When I first met Gracyn, her chances for survival were slim. Her heart was so badly damaged that using an experimental Berlin Heart became our only c⋯ As she awoke from her first surgery I was touched deeply by h⋯ spirituality. As we attended to her care over the nex⋯ mination, and sweet spirit inspired many of ⋯ heart surgeon. She is a remarkable little girl a⋯ touch your heart.

– Mark S. Bleiweis, M.D.
Director, Congenital Heart Cente⋯ ⋯ UF

Gracyn's Song reminds me of my own personal battles with disease and disability. This family's story invites us to face our struggles and—together—believe that our own songs have positive endings. A long time in the hospital. A family facing the unknown. Parents and brothers wondering what will happen to Gracyn. Honesty and doubts. Uncertainty and faith. Surgery, recovery, and hope: God was singing in each season, each question, each experience. So many people are hurting in today's world. Are you one of us? Read, sing, and experience this song. *Gracyn's Song* is a book we need. Join in and sing the song of hope with Gracyn and her family.

—**Chris Maxwell**
Author, Pastor, Director of Spiritual Life
www.chrismaxwellweb.com

As their pastor I've watched the DenBesten family weather this storm, with humility, tears, and patient endurance. God has used the faith of His child to impact many lives in our congregation and beyond. Through her faith, Gracyn has become a miraculous testimony to God's healing power. One of the highlights of my 34 years in ministry was worshipping with Gracyn as she sang on Father's Day, 2009. *Gracyn's Song* is a powerful reminder that God is still in the miracle business. This book will touch your heart, strengthen your faith, and help guide you through the storms of this life.

—**Dr. David Uth**
Senior Pastor, First Baptist Church of Orlando

I have been honored to participate in just a small way in Gracyn's story and can testify that her story is one of grace, faithfulness, healing, and joy. Soon after her heart transplant Gracyn joined me on stage to sing "Healer." As she lifted her voice, it was apparent she wasn't just singing a song but testifying to the truth that Jesus is indeed our healer and He is all we need. I'm grateful she has told her story in this book so that we can all learn from this sweet girl.

—**Kari Jobe**
Worship Leader, Recording artist

A valuable pastoral care resource, this book offers a rare view into one family's honest grappling with the distinctive issues of long-term medical crisis. Their journey from Gracyn's initial trauma through the spiraling stages of grief and ultimately into a new place of peace is, indeed, a beautiful song. Its melody is supported by the strong chords of a deep faith that trusts God with the full range of their frustration, doubt, anger, love, joy, and hope. I would especially recommend this engaging story to healthcare chaplains, pastoral care providers, and ministry students working with anticipatory grief in family systems.

—Lisa Jeffcoat
M.A.T., M.Div. Yale University Divinity School '03
Hospice (2004-2005); Hospital Chaplaincy (2007)

A crisis can be a puzzle. Where is God? What do we do? Why? This miraculous story is a gripping saga of a family that is suddenly thrown into a crisis. They survived that valley and the lessons they learned have been turned into a riveting book of hope. This book is an excellent resource of practical help for pastors, chaplains, counselors, caregivers, and for all who find themselves with their backs to the wall. *Gracyn's Song* is one of the most inspiring stories I have encountered in my 50 years of ministry.

—Dr. Jim Henry
Southern Baptist Convention President, 1994-1996

Gracyn's Song is powerful and transformational. Kris, Robin, and Gracyn open their hearts and allow the reader to walk with them through fears, questions, delights, and victories. As a counselor, I often work with others who are seeking wisdom for navigating through painful, unexpected, or frightening circumstances. *Gracyn's Song* will give them fuel for their journey because it is real—an open and beautiful picture of one family experiencing more than they could have imagined. Christ's power shines brightly through this story, not just because of the miraculous outcome, but because the DenBestens kept seeking Him through each step. For this reason, it will deeply impact the lives of readers, whether they are walking through a treacherous storm or just needing to connect with God's mighty hand through a beautiful journey.

—Holly Rockefeller, M.A.
Licensed Mental Health Counselor

GRACYN'S SONG

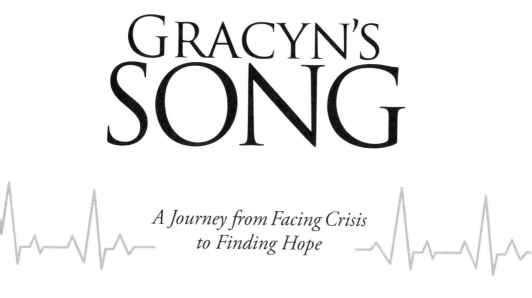

*A Journey from Facing Crisis
to Finding Hope*

KRIS & GRACYN DENBESTEN

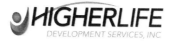

DEVELOPMENT SERVICES, INC

Oviedo, Florida

Gracyn's Song: A Journey from Facing Crisis to Finding Hope
By Kris DenBesten and Gracyn DenBesten

Published by HigherLife Development Services, Inc.
400 Fontana Circle
Building 1 Suite 105
Oviedo, FL 32765
(407) 563-4806
www.ahigherlife.com

ISBN 13: 978-1-935245-37-7
ISBN 10: 1-935245-37-6

Cover Design: r2cdesign—Rachel Lopez

First Edition
10 11 12 13 — 9 8 7 6 5 4 3 2 1
Printed in the United States of America

DEDICATION

This book is dedicated to the medical professionals who selflessly gave of themselves to care for Gracyn. Despite their own personal struggles and crises, they compassionately served our family day and night in our time of great need.

This book is also dedicated to the thousands who prayed, and continue to pray, for our family. Your prayers mean more to us than you will ever know. We are so thankful for each of you.

Finally, for those of you who are facing a crisis, or have faced one in the past, this book is for you. I pray that it will be an encouragement and a faith-builder for you as you walk through this time of trial.

Contents

PART ONE:
FACING THE CRISIS

PART TWO:
FACING THE UNKNOWN

PART THREE:
FACING THE LONG HAUL

CONTENTS

Visit **www.gracyn.org** for video, pictures, and more.

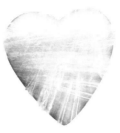

INTRODUCTION

It seems everywhere I turn these days people are hurting. Perhaps it's my advancing age. But I can't recall a time when I have known so many people dealing with a critical health crisis. Because of economic downturn, some face the crises of foreclosure, joblessness, and loss of hope. These are indeed tough times in which we are living. We never know what crisis the person sitting next to us could be enduring. My goal in sharing my family's story of facing a medical crisis with our nine-year-old daughter is to encourage others who are facing their own crises and fearing the unknown.

I'm not a counselor, clergy member, or medical professional. I'm simply a dad and husband whose family has a miraculous story. Faith, hope, and love carried us through a traumatic experience. It is my sincere desire that our story will encourage and guide you through your own time of crisis, whatever it may be.

While putting our story in book form, I have tried to keep it in chronological order as much as possible. The beginning chapters and ending chapters are true to the timeline in which they occurred. The middle chapters, however, are written around themes through which I seek to provide practical suggestions for those facing similar challenges.

In most chapters, there are entries from our family's journal we posted regularly on our Caring Bridge website (www.caringbridge. org/visit/gracyndenbesten). The edited journal entries in this book usually contain much raw emotion; they were written as updates while in the midst of our storm. It is noted when these entries were written by Gracyn, my wife, Robin, my sons, Cole and Brooks, and by me. Also, most chapters have a section at the end entitled "From Gracyn's Heart," which was dictated to me by my now ten-year-old daughter. In these sections, Gracyn is giving her perspective of what transpired.

Our family's story is told from our perspective of life, a Christian worldview that is tied to a deeply rooted, personal faith in Jesus Christ. I have included Scripture that helped our family process and make it through these tough times. Even if you do not share our faith perspective, I hope you will read this book for the encouragement it can provide.

A basic tenet of the Christian faith is God sending His only Son to redeem the world. Through Jesus's life, death, and resurrection, God provides the Way for all who believe in Jesus to receive eternal life. Regardless of how dark, dreary, or dire our current situation may be, we need not feel trapped by hopelessness. Our current circumstances do not determine our future or diminish our hope. God is in control and offers hope to all who believe. I have believed in Him for many years. But only recently I discovered what it really means to live by faith.

In the midst of our crisis, our good friends Todd and Melisa Setsma provided a strong example of individuals living by faith. They, too, endured a medical crisis. Jameson Setsma, their third son, was born July 13, 2008, with a rare skin disease called epidermolysis bullosa, or EB. Children with EB, which causes blisters to form all over their bodies, are often referred to as "butterfly children" because their skin is as fragile as a butterfly's wings.

On March 3, 2009, God healed Jameson by calling him to heaven to live in the Light. His short time on this earth is the most powerful testimony of faith, hope, and love I have ever encountered. God used this child to touch more lives in seven months than many of us will touch in a lifetime.

The faith of his family has inspired many. Our dear friends have endured great pain in this journey. Yet, their faith, hope, and love shine through them as a powerful testimony to the One who now holds their baby boy in His lap. Jameson has earned his reward. He has received his "well done." He is healed perfectly as he rests in the arms of his Lord and Savior Jesus Christ. We are blessed to have known this child of God. For us, his life and legacy account for so much.

Initially it may appear there are two completely different earthly outcomes to our respective families' crises. However, through faith, we know God miraculously answered both our families' prayers for healing: one child healed here on earth and the other in heaven.

The testimony of Jameson and the Setsma family strengthened my own faith and the faith of my family. In the midst of our crisis, when we needed to see faith with our own eyes, we looked at their example. For that I am, and will remain, eternally grateful.

We continually remember before our God and Father your work produced by faith, your labor prompted by love, and your endurance inspired by hope in our Lord Jesus Christ. (1 Thess. 1:3)

It is my hope and prayer that in reading our story your faith will be escalated and you will find encouragement, practical thoughts, and spiritual testimony that will empower you with the faith, hope, and love needed to carry you through any crisis you may face.

PART ONE

FACING THE CRISIS

*For video, pictures, and interviews that relate
to Part One, go to www.gracyn.org.*

CHAPTER 1

WHEN CRISIS CRUSHES YOU

FROM EARLIEST CHILDHOOD, GRACYN has been a singer at heart. By the age of two, she would stand on coffee tables and sing "God Bless America" in perfect pitch for anyone who would listen. She has always loved to sing, be it in church, at school, around the neighborhood, or blasting out karaoke hits from her room. She makes up many songs too—both silly kid songs and more serious songs of faith. Her mom and I have always known that the Lord has put a song in Gracyn's heart. She comes most fully alive as she shares her songs with others.

THE CRISIS BEGAN

Our entire family was eagerly looking forward to Christmas 2008. The approaching Christmas Eve was going to be extra special for us. Our youngest son, Brooks, was to be baptized, and his sister, Gracyn, was to sing a solo during the Christmas Eve service at our church.

The weekend before Christmas, Gracyn was not feeling well. She wanted to make sure she got better quickly so she could sing her song on Christmas Eve. By Monday she was still sick. Her mother, Robin, took her to the doctor. There they assumed she had a bug that was going around, gave her a breathing treatment, and prescribed an antibiotic. They foresaw her being fine in a few days.

The next couple of days, Gracyn appeared sluggish and extremely restless. Her breathing became labored. She had trouble sleeping and would not eat anything. We continued antibiotics and breathing treatments, and tried to persuade her to eat something. We assumed her lack of energy was related to her lack of nourishment.

At 3:00 a.m. the morning before Christmas, I was awakened by Gracyn standing at my bedside. Lifting the covers, I allowed her to slide in bed next to me. I don't remember her saying anything; however, the moment she put her hands on my back I became fully conscious. Her hands were freezing! Not giving it much thought, I suggested she put socks on her hands so they wouldn't be so cold if she rubbed them up against me again.

I had no idea what was really happening.

After a restless night, Gracyn was feeling so weak she could not muster the strength needed to climb out of bed.

"I think I should take her back to the doctor right now," Robin told me.

I agreed and carried Gracyn to the car, buckling her in for a trip to her pediatrician's office.

Thirty minutes later, Robin called. "We are in the ambulance headed to Arnold Palmer Hospital. Can you meet us there?" I could sense the urgency in her voice.

Surprised, I asked, "What's the problem?"

"I'm not sure," Robin said, "but they think she should be looked at there. She is so weak and lackadaisical. She may have a case of pneumonia or something."

As I drove to the hospital, I kept thinking Gracyn would be so disappointed if she wasn't able to sing her song. Upon arrival I was surprised to be greeted at the emergency room door by a very nice lady who asked, "Are you Mr. DenBesten?"

When I said yes, she asked that I follow her to where they had assigned Gracyn. As I followed the lady, my impression was that this hospital has outstanding customer service to meet me at the door like that. I figured they did that for everyone.

The seriousness of the situation didn't set in until I stepped into the room and noticed the grave looks on the faces of the doctor and three nurses working on my daughter. They were intently focused on finding a vein in her arm from which they could draw blood and in which to place an IV line. A hospital chaplain introduced himself and offered his support. Clouds of confusion rained down on me.

The next moments are a blur. Everything happened so quickly. Dr. Clark, the attending ER physician, took Robin and me aside. With a somber concern in his eyes, he informed us our daughter was critically ill. "We are all in agreement that her heart is failing," he said.

We were shocked! Anguish and fear flooded in on us as we tried to comprehend what was happening. We asked, "Her heart? She's only nine years old. She has always been the perfect picture of health. How in the world could this be happening?"

My mind flashed back to the feeling of Gracyn's cold hands on my back. Her cold hands and feet were the results of very low blood circulation to the extremities of her body. I was pierced with the realization my daughter had actually been dying right next to me earlier that morning. How could I have missed that? Her frozen hands were a distress warning. All I had done was cover them up so I could get some sleep. Guilt, fear, and desperation welled up inside me.

Gracyn was exhausted and scared. Informing her of what needed to happen, Robin and I tried to remain calm and positive. We explained to Gracyn that she probably would be spending a few days in the hospital. Nearly listless at this point, she was disappointed with this news but took it in stride.

A short time later, Dr. Nykanen, a knowledgeable and compassionate cardiologist, took us into a small, private room to inform us of the severity of Gracyn's situation. Compassionately, he explained that a virus had attacked our daughter's heart. Her heart was functioning at only twenty-percent of its capacity. She had a condition called viral myocarditis. What the doctor gave as the prognosis rocked our world: only one-third of the people who contract viral myocarditis will heal from it (if it is not too severe), one-third need to have a heart transplant, and the other third die from heart failure. We were mortified.

As Dr. Nykanen explained some of the potential procedures Gracyn needed, a sense of sickness, deep despair, and denial overwhelmed Robin and me. These procedures sounded drastic and painful. All was so sudden, frightening, and confusing. Realizing this was life-changing news, we were overcome with anticipatory grief.

"Not our little girl! This can't be happening! How could she possibly endure the pain of such procedures? If we could only change places with her," we kept saying to each other.

We began to pray instinctively, crying out to God for a miracle. We prayed she would be in the good-outcome group, who eventually heal from this vicious attack on the heart. We prayed for her to be spared of the frightening procedures that could be ahead of her. We prayed and prayed like never before.

Initially, it looked as though our prayers were being answered. Gracyn seemed to stabilize in response to the medication and oxygen they had given her. Being a determined little fighter, Gracyn put on a great act to convince everyone she was feeling much better. In fact, by early evening, she said she felt well enough to see some guests—her best friend, Grace, and her brothers, Cole and Brooks. She appeared to be rallying, which greatly encouraged us.

When doing their rounds around seven o'clock, the doctors asked if we could step out for an hour or so. Robin took this opportunity to spend some time with our boys. She rode home with my parents and the boys. They rounded up some clothes and essentials for the indefinite amount of time our boys would need to spend at their grandparents' house.

About an hour later, while Robin was still away, the medical staff summoned me to Gracyn's room as she was growing increasingly uneasy. Sensing her fear, I grabbed her hand in an attempt to console her. She courageously mustered a slight smile and asked where her mommy was. When I explained, Gracyn asked me to call Robin and tell her to come quickly.

Immediately I called Robin. "Gracyn's demeanor is taking a turn," I explained. "She really wants you here. Please, come quickly."

In the meantime, I did my best to calm down Gracyn, but it was of no use. She was extremely frightened and distressed. (Later Gracyn told me she thought she was going to die and desperately wanted both her mom and me to be there with her when that happened.)

THE CRISIS ESCALATED

Robin arrived just as the doctors determined Gracyn was not getting enough oxygen and needed to be placed on a respirator. As they began to prepare her for that procedure, Robin and I experienced a horror that hopefully few parents will ever experience: Gracyn became increasingly restless, agitated, and delirious (due to lack of oxygen).

At one point, her eyes rolled back in her head, and she began screaming, "I'm going to die!"

Sheer terror enveloped us. Robin and I became helpless spectators as our little girl fought valiantly for her life. Seeing our precious child endure such depths of pain and despair was pure torture. The fear of losing her paralyzed us as the brutal battle played out before our eyes. Completely powerless to join this fight, we could only pray and hope for the best.

In the midst of this horror, the doctors asked us to step out so they could perform the procedure to put Gracyn on the ventilator. Apprehensive, Robin and I retreated to the waiting room where friends and family comforted and prayed with us.

The doctors informed us they would need to put Gracyn on a heart-and lung-bypass ECMO machine. They explained this machine would allow her heart and lungs to rest and sustain her through the night. While on the ECMO machine, she would be heavily sedated, and her body paralyzed. In essence, she would be placed in a coma. Nearly everything we had prayed so fervently to avoid seemed to be taking place.

At that moment, it felt as though God was absent and turning a deaf ear to my cries. I asked, "Where are You, God? Why aren't You listening?" I have never felt so helpless, so alone, so emotionally depraved.

Eventually, our physicians informed us, "There's nothing you can do here tonight. It's critical for you to get as much rest as possible." They advised us to go home for the night and get some rest.

Robin and I reluctantly followed their advice. Exhausted, we ventured home in the early morning hours.

After arriving home, we soon found ourselves in Gracyn's bedroom. It was exactly how she'd left it, but the feel of the room was of absolute emptiness. I yearned to hug my little girl. Tears streamed down Robin's face as her hand gently stroked the comforter on Gracyn's bed. The empty room was filled with the fear that she may not return.

Lifting the Bible from her nightstand, I began to read Psalm 91. "He who dwells in the shelter of the Most High will rest in the shadow of the Almighty." By now I could barely speak as my emotions battled my voice. "I will say of the LORD, 'He is my refuge and my fortress, my God, in whom I trust.'" The next verse barely audible I choked and labored on, "Surely he will save you from the fowler's snare and from the deadly pestilence."

I collapsed on Gracyn's bed and wept uncontrollably. Robin and I cried until there were no more tears and prayed until we were out of words. With all that was left in us, we begged for God to bring Gracyn home to sleep in this bed once again. The desolate feelings stoked a desire to be near our boys. In the early morning, Robin and I drove to my parents' house to be with them when they would wake up. Later, while lying in total darkness on a bed in my parent's guest room, I thought, *What kind of way is this to spend Christmas?* There had been no baptism for Brooks or singing by Gracyn in church. The light in my life seemed to have gone dark. The joy in my heart had been covered up by grief. The presents under the tree held no meaning whatsoever. As the rising sun slowly displaced the darkness, it did nothing to dispel my sense of emptiness inside. I just wanted my little girl to come home.

When our boys woke up, they were surprised to see us. Their beaming faces warmed our hearts. It felt great to hold them tightly in our arms. Fighting to hold it together, we gently explained their sister was very sick and would need to be in the hospital for a while. After a brief, early-morning Christmas "celebration," we were back en route to the hospital.

As we entered her room that Christmas morning, I will never forget what I saw, heard, and thought. Gracyn lay sedated, paralyzed, and hooked up to countless devices and IV medications. Three medical professionals hovered over her as she (sustained only by life-support equipment), lay seemingly lifeless. The sounds were sobering: monitors beeping, machines rumbling, and nurses urgently relaying stats. The gravity of this scene broke my heart. Countless, unthinkable thoughts bombarded my mind: *She'll never get better. She's already gone. This is your fault. Remember all the bad things you've done? Well, this is your punishment.* Fear and anguish filled my mind with lies and left me with little resolve to combat these untruths.

Life was out of control. I had no idea what to do next. My whole world was in total chaos.

REFLECTION: Know God is with you.

In the midst of my utter despair, God stepped into my chaos. His nearness momentarily eased my fear. He replaced the desperate lies with truth. He reminded me that if I would fear only the Lord, there would be no reason for me to fear anything else. His presence would fulfill my greatest need.

> *In the fear of the LORD one has strong confidence, and one's children will have a refuge.* (Prov. 14:26 NRSV)

Feeling the sense of God's presence filled my thoughts with hope. It was as if God were speaking directly to my soul saying, "*My son, I am here with you; trust Me with this one.*"

I clearly recalled a statement from a dear friend a few years before. "Sometimes we don't fully understand that Jesus is all we need until we realize that Jesus is all we've got." At that very moment, for the first time, I realized my faith in Jesus Christ was all I had for dealing with this crisis. He was not absent, but right there with me. My faith in Christ proved critical throughout our crisis. Each time I began to feel abandoned, I believed—by faith—God was with me and that He was all I needed.

Everything became quiet and peaceful inside of me as God led my mind to focus on the very first Christmas morning and how

Christ had entered the world. It dawned on me that Jesus did not enter the world in joyful, peaceful surroundings. Instead, the Son of God arrived in the midst of utter chaos to oppressed, struggling parents who were not in their own home but in unfamiliar, chaotic surroundings—an animal shelter.

Jesus came into the world in the midst of utter crisis that first Christmas morning.

> *The virgin will be with child and will give birth to a son, and they will call him Immanuel—which means, "God with us."* (Matt.1:23)

And it was then I realized God—this same "Immanuel, 'God with us'"—was with Gracyn and me in the same way: in the midst of all our chaos on this Christmas morning. There was great comfort in knowing, beyond a shadow of a doubt, God was there with us as we faced this crisis. We were not alone. The Truth was with us. God was with us. Immanuel would strengthen us for what we were facing and whatever else would come our way.

> *And surely I am with you always, to the very end of the age.* (Matt. 28:20b)

FROM GRACYN'S HEART...

This was the scariest day in my life. I knew I was really sick, but I didn't know how badly. At first I just wanted to sing at church and be home for Christmas. Then it got very scary. I was so afraid that I was going to die. I asked for my mom and dad. However, my nurse said they couldn't be in my room while the doctors were doing their rounds. I started to feel like I was going to die. I just wanted to make sure my mom and dad were there with me. When my dad came in, I really thought it might be the last time I would see him. I was glad to see my mom, but I was scared and hurting by then.

When it got really bad, I got a strong feeling God was with me. It seemed like very bad things were happening around me, but I was comforted on the inside. It was like my body was at the hospital, but my soul was with God.

WHEN YOU ARE LOSING CONTROL OF YOUR LIFE

I PRAY DAILY FOR MY children: their future, health, safety, and other things. While I would love to tell you these prayers are always heartfelt, sometimes they are just repetitive, superficial requests I hurriedly make to God. Over the years, however, some of my most sincere conversations with God concerning my kids have been when articulating my greatest fear that something bad would happen to one of my children. Many times I have begged God to spare me of this heartbreak.

This Christmas morning, I was facing my worst fear head on. As my parental control was slipping away, my prayer life was about to enter a new dimension.

LOSING MY GRIP

Gracyn's heart had become so swollen it could no longer adequately pump blood through her body. Because of this, a large blood clot had formed in the left ventricle of her heart. This presented another grave danger: if this clot were to break free, it could cause massive injury or even death.

As Gracyn lay motionless—sustained only by life support equipment—the medical team began to explain to me the workings of the ECMO machine. The surgeons had placed a cannula (tube) into a large vein in Gracyn's neck to withdraw her blood prior to its reaching her heart. Her blood was being circulated outside her body through this machine, where it was oxygenated and warmed before being returned through her neck to an artery, which would carry the blood throughout her body. This was a terrifying sight. Making a morbid sound, the ECMO machine substituted for Gracyn's heart and lungs and allowed them to rest in hope they could possibly heal. We were warned the process could be damaging to her other organs—especially her kidneys and her liver—and increase the risk for blood clots and other complications.

Seeing Gracyn's blood pumping through this machine and hearing of the potential risks were just too much for us to handle. We were in shock, struggling to process it all. Robin and I had to make a choice: freak out and lose it, or remain calm and seek God in prayer. By His grace, God provided us with the strength to choose the latter.

We paused and began to pray about our worst fears and anxieties. We thanked God for this intimidating machine and prayed for its effectiveness to be proven out. We expressed our deep gratitude for the caring and knowledgeable people who were attending our daughter. As we earnestly asked God for His help, we were comforted by a calming sense of peace.

Without a doubt, this precious time of prayer prepared our hearts and minds for what we were about to hear. Soon afterwards the doctors dropped the biggest bombshell of all on us: "There is really nothing more we can do for Gracyn. There is no medicine or procedure that will make her better. All we can do is sustain her life for a time with the hope her body will heal itself."

With a serious look and through compassionate words, Dr. Nykanen began explaining the likelihood of Gracyn's need for a heart transplant. My head dizzied as my body reached the point of emotional overload. Robin and I could not begin to comprehend all that was happening. Up until that point, a heart transplant and death seemed like one and the same to us. They had been two options we could not bring ourselves to consider.

We were losing our grip on our daughter's life. Her well-being and future were beyond our control. While hearing all this bad news, our parental instincts were screaming for us to step up and do something. Daddies are supposed to protect their little girls. We're wired to jump in and be the hero. Mommies want to hug their precious angels and console them. However, Robin and I were rendered powerless to aid our suffering child. There was nothing we could do.

For just a moment, I began to doubt God and question why He would let something like this happen. *How could the purest heart I know of be under such an attack? Why would God allow this to happen to one of His children? Didn't He know how much Gracyn loves Him?* I began to feel sorry for myself. Anger and doubt welled up inside me. With all my strength, I was struggling to hold on. I had reached the end of my rope.

STRENGTHENING GOD'S GRIP

The battle for my faith raged as I fought feelings of hopelessness. I was descending into the depths of depression. It was then a short Bible verse—one that would continually play an important role throughout this battle—came into my mind: "Be still and know that I am God" (Ps. 46:10). It was as though God Himself were whispering reassuring words in my ear!

This verse provided the framework for realigning my thoughts and actions. With those few words He breathed peace in the midst of my anxiety and calmed my anger, despair, and other raging emotions. Through "being still" I was reminded God is in control. Through acknowledging He alone is God I was able to relinquish my heavy load to Him. The crisis still remained. But God lifted me up from despair. He would carry me through—despite my heavy load—if I would just trust Him. I resolved to grow in faith regardless of the outcome.

Robin and I agreed that God was, in fact, our only hope. Trusting in Him and His faithfulness was our sole option. There was nothing more we—out of our own strength and resources—could do. We had reached the point of knowing only God could do this.

It was at this point our faith in God became the most real kind of faith. We chose to trust God and surrender every ounce of control to Him. We began to pray and trust God like never before. We knew—as in, "be still and know"—God was in control of this crisis. We realized that when the doctors were saying there was nothing more they could do, God was saying He could do all things. Gracyn's life was no longer in human hands, but in His.

Do not be anxious about anything, but in everything, by prayer and petition, with thanksgiving, present your requests to God. And the peace of God, which transcends all understanding, will guard your hearts and your minds in Christ Jesus. (Phil. 4:6-7)

I still needed another aspect of surrendering my grip and seeking to strengthen God's grip in my life: asking others to pray for me and my family. I don't know if it was pride or just a desire for privacy, but I had never been the type to ask others to pray for me. I believed in prayer and had prayed many prayers for others. However, up to this point, I had always felt as though prayer for me was just something between God and me. I did not comprehend how much I needed the prayers of others. This crisis of faith brought the realization that asking others to pray for us is actually an act of obedience. It is a way of proclaiming our faith in God. Armed with this truth, I began asking everyone I could think of to intercede in prayer for Gracyn and my family.

Over the next few days, we literally survived on prayer. People by the thousands were praying. First, our pastor asked nearly six thousand people who attended our church's Christmas Eve services (at which Gracyn was supposed to sing) to pray for us. Then e-mails, phone calls, and text messages all went out calling for prayer for our little girl. Eventually, we discovered the wonderful Caring Bridge website where we journaled about Gracyn's situation. Through that website, thousands more joined in prayer. Over time, our Caring Bridge site received over half million hits. We were amazed at all who began to step in on our behalf to pray for Gracyn and to strengthen our faith. The power of prayer became increasingly evident in our lives. A couple of weeks into our journey, I posted this on our website:

FROM MY JOURNAL...

January 11, 2009

I cannot begin to fathom facing something like this without faith. I know we could not handle this on our own. We are sustained by the power of God's mighty hand and lifted by the prayers and support of the body of Christ. Many have questioned whether they could show the strength of faith that Gracyn, Robin, and I are apparently revealing. In the past, I would have questioned this myself. Yet, today I can assure everyone that if you place all your trust in God you, too, will find the measure of faith that can move mountains. There is an amazing dose of strength and peace waiting for each of us at the point of realizing that only God can do this. When we reach that point of recognizing Jesus is all we've got, it's then we can fully appreciate that Jesus is all we need.

As Robin and I focus on the Most High, we will rest in the shadow of the Almighty and walk confidently in faith that our God will move this mountain. We understand it won't be easy and know we aren't exempt from the pain. However, we are empowered by the assurance that God is with us wherever we go.

If you would, please, simply pray that our faith will be escalated. Pray that Gracyn and the rest of us will continue to walk closer and closer with our God as we trust Him to lift us, uphold us, and to cultivate us physically, mentally, and spiritually. The Lord is our Shepherd. We are His sheep. He is all we need.

Through this experience, Robin and I have learned the true meaning of prayer is surrendering our control to God. In doing so, it helped us look beyond ourselves and our crisis and focus on God and His power. It has brought others together with us in a supportive and effective community of faith. God's powerful grip on our lives has been strengthened.

REFLECTION: RELEASE YOUR BURDEN TO GOD.

Handing over the control of our crisis and its outcome to the One who made and governs the universe was both humbling and reassuring. Through prayer we were able to show our total dependence and complete trust in our God. We had to release our tight grip of this burden in order to place it securely in His omnipotent hands.

While passing through this insane crisis, we thought about the familiar story of Abraham and his beloved son Isaac. Isaac meant more to Abraham than anyone or anything on earth. Surprisingly, God tells Abraham to sacrifice his son on an altar. As crazy as this command sounds, Abraham obeyed God and put his trust in Him:

> When they came to the place that God had shown him, Abraham built an altar there and laid the wood in order. He bound his son Isaac, and laid him on the altar, on top of the wood. Then Abraham reached out his hand and took the knife to kill his son. But the angel of the LORD called out to him from heaven, and said, "Abraham! Abraham!" And he said, "Here I am." He said, "Do not

lay your hand on the boy or do anything to him; for now I know that you fear God, since you have not withheld your son, your only son, from me." (Gen. 22:9-12 NRSV)

What a perplexing story! How could a parent completely trust God in that way? The example of Abraham's faith helped us. Like Abraham, we had to unequivocally trust in the goodness of God and place our child's life in His hands, regardless of the circumstance. As much as we loved our daughter, we realized God loves her even more. She is His, not ours.

As difficult as it was, Robin and I resolutely handed over our beloved Gracyn to the God of our fathers. While we continuously prayed He would return her to us, we had an unshakable peace and ability to accept God's will. Regardless of the outcome, she belonged in His hands.

Humble yourselves, therefore, under God's mighty hand, that he may lift you up in due time. Cast all your anxiety on him because he cares for you. (1 Pet. 5:6-7)

FROM GRACYN'S HEART...

I don't remember being on the ECMO machine because I was so sick at the time. (I did see a baby on ECMO while I was at Shands, and the machine looked really creepy and scary.) I still have scars on my neck where they hooked up the machine. (Whenever I lie down, I always try to cover the scar with a blanket or with my hair.) I do thank God for that machine, though, because it helped save my life.

Prayer is such an awesome thing because when we pray we get to talk to a real God who listens and who can do anything. I'm so thankful for all the people who prayed for me. I couldn't have made it through everything without prayer—my own prayers and the prayers of many others. Whenever I would get scared or sad, I would always pray. God always gave me strength to go on. When we pray, we show God how much we trust Him. I know He likes that.

CHAPTER 3

WHEN YOU STRUGGLE WITH "WHY?"

A S PARENTS, ROBIN AND I battled guilt as we wondered why all this had happened: *How could we have prevented it? Why hadn't we taken Gracyn to the hospital sooner?* Gracyn's cardiologist, Dr. Nykanen, continually reassured us we had done nothing wrong, nor could we have done anything to prevent this from happening.

Viral myocarditis, the viral condition that had attacked Gracyn's heart, is a very rare diagnosis. In fact, viral myocarditis occurs in less than one percent of viral infection cases. Yet, in young adults it accounts for up to twenty percent of all sudden-death cases. It occurs when any common virus, which normally passes through the body and renders cold-like symptoms, inexplicably takes an aggressive tract to the heart. As the body's immune system tries to wipe out the virus, it actually damages the heart, causes inflammation, and weakens the heart's ability to function properly.

There usually is no answer to these *why-did-all-this-happen* questions. Dr. Nykanen encouraged us to clear our minds from wondering why so we could fully focus on what we would need to do as our next steps in this process.

Asking the "Why?" Question

As Gracyn's condition continued to decline, Dr. Nykanen was always encouraging and careful not to diminish our hope. However, his conversations were now directed towards Gracyn's need of a heart transplant. He explained the type of ECMO machine being used to keep Gracyn alive was only capable of sustaining her for 7-10 days before major complications would occur. Already her body had begun to shut down. Her kidneys and liver were declining rapidly. The blood clots were of major concern. Tests showed her heart was actually weakening rather than improving.

A Berlin Heart®—an experimental artificial heart for kids that could keep Gracyn alive while she awaited a heart transplant—was being discussed with us by Dr. Nykanen. Gracyn would need to be transferred to Shands Hospital at the University of Florida in Gainesville, over one hundred miles away. A teaching and research hospital, Shands had doctors and nurses who were experienced with the Berlin Heart®, and therefore, Shands would be the best place for Gracyn based on her condition.

Robin and I hated to leave the familiar surroundings of our hometown hospital. A great sense of trust and comfort had been built by Gracyn's caregivers. She had received excellent care from the medical team. These professionals had given their best to save and sustain Gracyn's life. We were comforted continually by many supporters who would visit, encourage us, and pray for Gracyn. The waiting room had become our refuge filled with friends, family, and community. A hospital is the worst possible place to spend the holidays, but at Arnold Palmer Hospital we were comfortable. We knew we were not alone.

Facing a transfer to Gainesville wasn't what we wanted. Going to Gainesville meant Gracyn was getting worse. It meant being away from home, having new doctors, dealing with the experimental Berlin Heart® machine, and ultimately, a heart transplant. We could not fathom one good thing about being transferred to Gainesville. Robin and I remained in constant prayer. We prayed God would work a miracle and heal Gracyn's heart. We begged God to not send us to Gainesville.

I asked my pastor, David Uth, to pray specifically that we would not need to go to Gainesville. He said, "Maybe God wants you in Gainesville. I get the distinct feeling God has some people he wants you to meet in Gainesville. There are doctors, nurses, and families there whom God wants you to impact. I believe He has a purpose for you to carry out while there."

That was not what I wanted to hear. On top of everything else we were going through, I could not comprehend why God would want us in Gainesville. I asked, "Why wasn't God answering our prayers? Why did this have to happen to my daughter? Why was everything going so wrong? Why? Why? Why?!"

For a brief time the *why* questions inflamed my anxiety and weakened my faith. They took my mind off God and what He could do and caused me to focus on myself. Instead of trusting in *what* God could do, I was worried about *why* this was happening to us. Fortunately, at some point in the midst of my asking *why*, God once again redirected my mind and spoke to my heart: *"Be still and know that I am God"* (Ps. 46:10).

That verse hit home. Something clicked! My perspective began to shift. God led me to process our crisis and all its unknowns in a different way. Rather than asking God *why*, I should, instead, start asking God *what*: "God, what are You going to do through this? What are You teaching me? What should I be praying for? What should I do next?"

As I began doing this my attitude rapidly improved. I accepted Gracyn's challenges as opportunities to receive God's guidance and to seek His plan. No longer could I be consumed by worry. My focus needed to shift from worrying about myself to aligning my actions with God's perfect plan.

Moving Beyond "Why?"

Gracyn's condition did not improve over the weekend. The decision was made for her to be transferred to Gainesville. Getting her there was a challenge. With all the machines, monitors, and IVs connected to Gracyn, a 100-mile drive on rough roads was out of the question. However, no one of Gracyn's age and size had ever been airlifted by helicopter while being sustained by an ECMO machine. They had transported babies, but never a nine-year-old. Doctors, logistic teams, and many others diligently worked to figure it out.

After hours of measuring, changing plans, and modifying equipment numerous times, the team determined that Gracyn would be transported to Gainesville in the largest medevac helicopter available in the southeastern United States by a Miami-based flight team. As she was wheeled by—still unconscious and unaware of anything that was transpiring—we stood and cheered. We cheered for her, the flight team, surgeon, and specialists who were accompanying her and necessary in the event something went wrong. We applauded the caregivers and hospital we were leaving behind. Most importantly, we exalted the Lord whom we were trusting to carry her through this time of great peril.

Robin and I were in no shape to drive. Our good friends, the McKees, volunteered to drive us to Gainesville. Robin tried unsuccessfully to nap in the backseat while I, trying my best not to be overwhelmed by the uncertainty that would lie ahead, rode up front with my friend, Matt.

I should have been losing it while helplessly monitoring my daughter's fight for life. Physically, I had not slept in days and had developed a serious sinus infection. Mentally, I found it impossible to think clearly about anything. Emotionally, I was in a battle of proportion never before imagined. What else could go wrong? It only kept getting worse. However, because I had surrendered to God's control of my life and circumstances—especially this crisis—spiritually, I was strengthened in spite of my weakness. God gave me the necessary courage to move ahead.

> *Have I not commanded you? Be strong and courageous. Do not be terrified; do not be discouraged, for the LORD your God will be with you wherever you go.* (Josh. 1:9)

Prayer and Scripture helped bring us to the point of believing anything could be endured and everything could be done with Christ's help.

> *I can do all things through Christ who strengthens me.* (Phil. 4:13 NKJV)

REFLECTION:
Seek what instead of why.

I have found many of our *why* questions cannot be answered in our limited understanding of God and His ways. We only know His ways are not our ways. His reason for *why* is not bound by earth or heaven, time or eternity.

> *"For my thoughts are not your thoughts, neither are your ways my ways," declares the LORD. "As the heavens are higher than the earth, so are my ways higher than your ways and my thoughts than your thoughts."* (Isa. 55:8-9)

Sometimes the answers to our *why* questions can only be answered by God. We needed to trust God and accept His ways even when we did not fully understand the *whys.*

> *Trust in the LORD with all your heart and lean not on your own understanding; in all your ways acknowledge him, and he will make your paths straight.* (Prov. 3:5-6)

I have begun to comprehend the *why* questions tend to weaken our faith, while the *what* questions help strengthen it. The *why* questions confuse us and distract our attention, whereas the *what* questions open our hearts and minds to receiving God's perfect provision.

> *My flesh and heart may fail, but God is the strength of my heart and my portion forever.* (Ps. 73:26)

As my prayer focused on asking God "*What?*" it opened my heart to receive the direction that only He can provide. I began to pray, "God, what do You want me to do next? What's that, God? Trust

You, rely fully on You, and get on up to Gainesville?…OK, I've got it, God! And I won't even think about asking *why."*

From Gracyn's Heart…

I didn't know why these really hard things were happening to me. Sometimes I would wonder and ask my parents, "Why do I have to be in a hospital? Why did this happen to me? Why does this have to be so hard on me? Why couldn't this have happened to someone else instead of me?"

I would always get sad when I thought about these things. It would make me feel like I was never going to get better. My dad wrote about one of those times in our Caring Bridge journal (Monday, February 23):

> *There are times Gracyn gets frustrated as her circumstance over-whelms her. Gracyn longs for home, for normalcy, and to be anywhere but stuck in this hospital…nothing unusual considering her situation. We usually let her cry a bit, get it all out, and then pray for God to restore hope and take away the pain. But this after-noon was different.*
>
> *Gracyn somewhat defiantly declined the opportunity to pray. Clearly distracted, she questioned why God would allow something like this to happen to her. She even doubted whether God really cared about her anyhow.*
>
> *Her mother and I clearly sensed the spiritual battle our daughter was facing. We explained some of our own struggles with the why questions and how we found the only solid defense for an attack like this is prayer. Robin and I each took a turn praying. There was a prolonged quiet as we silently prayed for Gracyn to release her anxiety to God. Soon tears welled in our eyes as she whimpered the*

most beautiful and humble prayer of repentance, love, and heart-felt petition to her Savior.

Today we experienced prayer as it is meant to be: the three of us enjoying the steadfast presence of our King, who was lifting Gracyn in love while restoring her faith and showering us with His grace.

I'm so glad God pulled my family and me through those tough times. He always loved me and had a plan for me. I just had to trust Him.

My advice to those who are going through similar hard times is to not get discouraged with worrying about all the *whys*. Instead, believe, pray, and trust that God has a plan.

PART TWO

FACING THE
UNKNOWN

*For video, pictures, and interviews that relate
to Part Two, go to www.gracyn.org.*

CHAPTER 4

WHEN YOU DON'T KNOW WHAT'S NEXT

GOING TO A NEW medical center and facing the many challenges brought us great anxiety. We'd never spent any time in Gainesville, much less Shands Hospital. We doubted the outstanding care Gracyn had received at Arnold Palmer could be duplicated anywhere else. The fear of the unknown was devastating. We had no clue what we were doing. We felt like helpless pawns being manipulated in some dramatic tragedy. We had no idea where we would eat or sleep, or what challenges we would find upon our arrival. We just knew our immediate destination was Gainesville, and we were dreading it.

GOD'S BEST PROVISION

As we walked into Shands Hospital for the first time, we were shocked by the stark difference between the new, state-of-the-art, privately funded children's hospital we had left in Orlando and the aging, university medical center for the general public in Gainesville. The cheery, kid-friendly entrance (designed and built by

Walt Disney World) to Arnold Palmer Hospital now was replaced with the shocking (almost scary) scene of numerous adult patients in hospital gowns—some connected to IV machines and monitors—loitering in the first floor lobby.

Stopping at the information desk, we were informed the PICU (Pediatric Intensive Care Unit) was on the tenth floor and probably where we would find Gracyn. Entering Arnold Palmer Hospital had been quite different. There it required signing in at a security desk and receiving a personal security tag before proceeding to any of the floors of the hospital. At Shands, the receptionist pointed to the elevator and told us to head on up.

Arriving on the tenth floor we found a phone and the instructions to call for entry to the PICU. We looked at one another and shrugged. I cautiously raised the receiver to my ear. Someone answered and confirmed Gracyn had arrived safely via helicopter and was being transferred from the transportable ECMO machine to one of Shands' ECMO units.

Eventually, a kind, young nurse named Stephanie—who soon became one of our favorite, most trusted caregivers—introduced herself. Stephanie informed us things were progressing smoothly. It was going to take a while before we could see Gracyn or her new doctors. We were instructed to find a seat in the waiting room, which resembled a small, poorly lit college dorm room. "Welcome to the University of Florida," my friend Matt light-heartedly joked as we decided to wait in the hallway instead.

While we waited, Robin and I were growing increasingly edgy and troubled. We felt like it had been an eternity since we had seen Gracyn. We were ill at ease in the unfamiliar surroundings…that is, until we saw the flight team and surgeon from Orlando walk by as they were departing for their helicopter. While we had only known these people for a very short time, they seemed like long lost friends. The transfer had gone well. Our hometown surgeon, Dr. DeCampli, encouraged us by saying, "I have a good feeling about this one."

I felt sick, scared, and completely exhausted as we first met the team overseeing the care of our daughter: Dr. Bleiweis (chief surgeon), Dr. Mulhotra (surgeon), and Dr. Fricker (chief cardiologist). The doctors could sense our apprehension as we gathered in the gloomy waiting room to hear what they had to say. Although our anxiety level was off the charts, suddenly a curious thing happened. Peace, much like we felt on Christmas morning, overwhelmed us. The more these doctors spoke, the more we realized God had gone before us and had chosen these men to use their knowledge, skills, and compassion to coordinate the healing process for our daughter. We recognized they were God's best provision for our daughter's critical need…and her parents' peace of mind.

Dr. Bleiweis explained the Berlin Heart® would be Gracyn's best hope for survival. This chief surgeon spoke of prior patients who had been sustained by the Berlin Heart® for up to nine months before receiving a successful heart transplant. Explaining that the experimental device had not yet been approved by the FDA and could only be used in cases where other alternatives were slim, Dr. Bleiweis was confident he could get one in for Gracyn.

The business man in me popped out, and I asked, "Since it's experimental, what if my insurance won't cover it?"

The doctor's response set the tone for what we would come to expect from this team: "Right now, I really don't care about that.

I am here to save your daughter's life. The Berlin Heart® represents the best avenue for me to accomplish that. We have a long history of doing the right things to save patients' lives here at Shands Hospital. That is my only priority. At some point, the business end of this may be discussed and worked out. Right now, you don't need to worry about that."

While we were not yet comfortable in our new surroundings, could not fully comprehend our circumstance, and had no idea what would come next, we knew after talking to these doctors that God had us exactly where we needed to be. Our fears, anxieties, and discomfort still existed. Yet, because we knew God was orchestrating the entire process, we found the courage and confidence to take the next step.

GOD'S PERFECT PLAN

Receiving the Berlin Heart® was a miracle itself. Manufactured in Germany, it has been used in Europe for a number of years. In 2007 the U.S. Food and Drug Administration granted conditional approval for the EXCOR pediatric Berlin Heart® device to be used in compassionate care cases for experimental testing to determine whether the FDA will eventually grant approval for use in the United States. Ours would be the fourth time the cardiac team at Shands would use the Berlin Heart® in an effort to save the life of a child.

As a result of his prior experience, commitment, and compassionate determination, Dr. Bleiweis was able to secure a Berlin Heart® for a quick delivery. We would later find out Dr. Bleiweis had to do some serious string-pulling to secure that Berlin Heart® for Gracyn. Because her situation was so dire, the likelihood for failure was extremely high. Regardless, Dr. Bleiweis, Shands HealthCare, and Berlin Heart, Inc. agreed to proceed despite the overwhelming risk.

Needless to say, we are extremely grateful to everyone who worked tirelessly behind the scenes to iron out the arrangements for Gracyn to receive this life-saving device. How amazing that God would go before us to bring all these people and cutting-edge technology together. He had worked out every detail for us. Shands Hospital in Gainesville, Florida, was exactly where God wanted us to be. And to think I had prayed so hard for us to stay in Orlando!

December 30 would be the day of Gracyn's surgery to install the Berlin Heart®. What an amazing machine. It is designed for medium- to long-term support for patients with failing hearts. The power unit is a three-hundred-pound, electric-powered, cart-mounted component that pumps air through two tethered lines connected to pumps sitting outside the body. As the figure (below) shows, cannulas (tubes) are inserted beneath the rib cage and intricately connected to the appropriate arteries and the patient's heart.

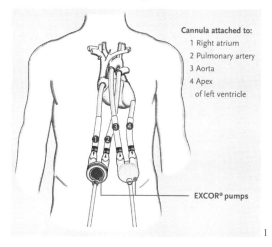

Cannula attached to:
1 Right atrium
2 Pulmonary artery
3 Aorta
4 Apex
of left ventricle

EXCOR® pumps

1

---

1 From www.berlinheart.de/englisch/patienten/EXCOR/Funktionsweise, 2010.

Blood is suctioned from the heart's right atrium through the tube to a VAD (ventricular assist device), which rests outside the stomach and pumps the blood back to the pulmonary artery where it enters the lungs. The lungs do the work of oxygenating the blood, which is suctioned back out through another tube to a second VAD that pumps it to the aorta with enough pressure to distribute it throughout the body. The Berlin Heart® practically functions as a human heart and allows the body to function properly because it is receiving blood in much the same way it would if the heart were working properly. The Berlin Heart® can sustain patients for many months while they await a donor heart.

Needless to say, this was very serious surgery. We had no idea what to expect. Yet we trusted God would work through the skill of our surgeons' hands and through the design of this remarkable life-saving machine. We were confident that this, indeed, was a part of His plan. The following is Robin's Caring Bridge post requesting prayer the night of Gracyn's surgery.

From Robin's journal...

Tuesday, December 30, 2008

Gracyn is on the list for a new heart. This will take time. Please pray specifically for:

1. No bleeding post-op. It is like walking a tightrope to manage her blood's consistency while she is on the Berlin Heart®. Pray the Lord gives wisdom to those overseeing this process.

2. Pray for healing of Gracyn's other organs. Her kidneys have suffered greatly throughout this ordeal and must heal before any transplant. Pray for her liver and lungs to heal as well.

3. Pray for the moment when Gracyn is aware enough to see she has a machine attached to her body. The doctors have told us this can be extremely hard on children. We couldn't warn her ahead of time. Pray the Lord will give us words to comfort her during this delicate time.

4. Pray for our boys and our family as we eventually discover what this means for our "normal" family life over the next few, days, weeks, and months.

5. Finally, because the Lord has shown me Gracyn will receive a heart—a heart He has always known of—I ask you to pray for the family of the child whose sweet heart will live in Gracyn. I pray for their peace, for their understanding, for their pain, for their loss, and, most importantly, for their salvation... that they may be reunited with their precious angel in heaven one day.

For those of you who don't know me, I like to plan. I like to have my ducks in a row. I like to think I can keep my life, and that of my family, nice and neat. It's just my nature.

"Father, I stand in awe of You this day. You have taught me so much over the last few days, hours, minutes. You've tried to teach me before to let go of the wheel and let You drive. Forgive me for taking it back from You over and over throughout this life. Forgive me for not fully trusting in You. Father, I give You the wheel now and trust You forever more. In so doing, I find faith like a child: the faith of a mustard seed. I rest quietly in Your arms of love. I wait upon You to direct my path and that of our family. You are mighty to save. Thank You for Your Word: 'Be still and know that I am God.' I finally get it, Lord. I stand in awe of You and what You are doing. To God be the glory!"

REFLECTION:
TRUST IN GOD'S LIFE-CHANGING POWER.

As our family faced impossible situations on unfamiliar turf with medical experts saying things we never imagined hearing, we had no idea what to expect. We felt so inadequate for the task before us. While we were thankful for our devoted family, wonderful friends, and incredible medical team, Robin and I had to process all that was happening and act prudently on our daughter's behalf. The task was daunting.

We could not have survived the short-term crises or the long-haul medical challenges apart from our faith in God and the power He gave us. I am not claiming we are some kind of spiritual giants. We are simply individuals who have been to the point of surrendering all our hopes, dreams, and desires for our daughter to the One who created, loves, and knows her better than anyone else.

We have found that God's Word is true: even small faith—as tiny as a mustard seed—yields incomparable power in the believer's life. This power is not found in the amount of faith, but in the power of God.

> *If you have faith as small as a mustard seed, you can say to this mountain, 'Move from here to there' and it will move. Nothing will be impossible for you.* (Matt. 17:20b)

By faith nothing seemed impossible when we waited on and listened to God. We could see Him at work—orchestrating every detail, taking care of all our true needs—right before our eyes. For that which we could not figure out, He already had a plan. For that which we had no resource within us to handle, God gave us His power.

It wasn't easy reaching this point of faith nor maintaining it. Many times throughout our journey, we would struggle when we found ourselves again and again facing the seemingly impossible. We would feel vulnerable and frightened to push ahead. However, in each crisis, through trusting in God's life-changing power, it became easier to know what to expect next. God would move any mountain in our way.

> *With human beings this is impossible, but with God all things are possible.* (Matt. 19:26b TNIV)

From Gracyn's Heart...

It was really hard living in the hospital because I never knew what was going to happen next. Sometimes scary things would happen with other kids. Then I would get worried that something bad would happen to me. I never knew if it was going to be a good day or a bad day because some days everything would be fine but then quickly would turn horribly bad.

I didn't know what to expect with the Berlin Heart®. I didn't know anybody who had been on one. It was pretty scary. My mom and dad would make me feel comfortable about it…and so would my nurses. (I really loved my nurses. They helped me get through so much.)

I am very thankful for Dr. Bleiweis. When I first met him right after I woke up from my Berlin surgery, I hugged him and told him I was one of God's miracles. I knew God had chosen Dr. Bleiweis to be part of those miracles. When I heard his name, I thought it sounded like Dr. Wise Eyes. So, that's what I called him for the rest of the time. I still call him that today. I think he kind of likes that name! I'm glad there are people like Dr Bleiweis because so many kids need his help. He is so smart, caring, and compassionate. When it comes to kids and hearts, he totally knows how to handle everything. I am very grateful for him. God uses him to help give kids a new chance at life.

I also am very thankful for Dr. Fricker, who takes care of me now, and all the great people who cared for me at Shands Hospital. They are the best! And, of course, I am thankful for the Berlin Heart®. God used a lot of people and a lot of things to help me get by. Most of all, I am thankful to God who makes all things possible!

CHAPTER 5

WHEN YOU ARE PRAYING
FOR A MIRACLE

WHEELING GRACYN IN FROM the operating room, Dr. Bleiweis, Dr. Mulhotra, and "Berlin Bob" (the Berlin Heart®, Inc. specialist) gave us the good news: Gracyn's surgery had gone extremely well. Her new lifeline, the Berlin Heart®, which we were seeing for the first time, had been successfully implanted. When he had placed the Berlin Heart® cannula into the left ventricle of Gray's heart, Dr. Bleiweis had carefully removed the large blood clot from that ventricle. "Berlin Bob" began explaining the Berlin Heart® to us. However, we were so overwhelmed by everything we could barely concentrate on a word he was saying. We were just grateful our daughter had survived the surgery. What a miracle!

FROM ROBIN'S JOURNAL...

Wednesday, December 31, 2008

Gray came through her surgery beautifully. The doctors let us see her last night around 11:00 p.m. She was already lifting her eyebrows trying to let us know she heard us. Her skin color was beautiful, and her body temp was perfect. She was already trying to breathe over the respirator. PRAISE GOD!

The Berlin pump is literally a miracle. I can't describe what it's like to see a machine standing in for your child's heart, allowing her to live. We've realized our Christmas miracle was the Lord's saving Gracyn's life Christmas Eve in Orlando. Thank You, Father. The second miracle was moving her successfully to Shands. The third was the availability and insertion of the Berlin Heart® Machine. The fourth is how well she did in surgery and how well she is responding today. God is in the business of making miracles...and I can't put into words how beautiful each one is.

Time passed slowly as we waited for the anesthesia and paralytic medicines to wear off, which, we were told, could take up to seventy-two hours. In time, Gracyn began opening and blinking her eyes. Eventually she was able to stare at us and slightly move her left hand. By later that evening, as I leaned over her bed, Gracyn clumsily reached up and brushed the goatee on my chin with her fingers. That brief touch seemed to reconnect me with my little girl. To me it was evidence she was still here. Her touch reached directly into my soul, reminding me of God's power to perform the miraculous.

The medical team wanted to see some movement of her right side and feet. Due to the rigid position of Gracyn's head while she was on the ECMO machine they had been unable to perform any testing of her brain activity. Now that she was on the Berlin Heart® and her head could move freely, an early morning CAT scan was ordered.

Not even realizing a new year had dawned—passing from 2008 to 2009—Robin and I eventually went to sleep that night.

Anticipate Battles

A sick feeling overwhelmed us as we entered Gracyn's room on New Year's Day. As Gracyn was lying asleep in her bed, it almost looked as though her torso was disconnected from her legs. A nurse kept prompting her to move her right foot over and over again. Gracyn was not waking up or moving at all.

Fearing Gracyn was paralyzed, Robin immediately became discouraged. A new terrifying thought began to fester: *You've been worried about her heart, but it's her brain that is the real concern.* The battle for our faith intensified as sick thoughts raced in and bombarded our minds.

Robin and I immediately huddled at Gracyn's bedside and began to pray. We knew what we were experiencing could be overcome only with prayer. "Be still and know I am God" (Ps. 46:10).

God began to ease our minds by once again reminding us that He is in control. As our prayers concluded, we were still a bit anxious, yet God once again sent His peace and lifted us with His strength. A song was rising from the CD player next to Gracyn's bed about praising God no matter what storm we may be facing. It was the perfect song at the perfect time. Robin and I glanced quick smiles at each other, confirming God's presence in our own storm.

Something truly amazing happened next. Gracyn awoke during this song and moved her left hand just enough to hold Robin's hand. We all began to weep with joy! God had graciously shown us His divine power through this victory. He also strengthened our faith so we might be better equipped to handle what we were about to face. About this time, Dr. Mulhotra asked us to meet with him in a private room. (As hospital veterans, we knew meetings in private rooms generally did not bring good news.)

"The CAT scan shows Gracyn suffered a stroke to the left frontal part of her brain probably from a blood clot breaking free," Dr. Mulhotra explained.

Her surgeon went on to explain some of the potential ramifications from this stroke. Gracyn's speech could be affected, or she may not be able to move the right side of her body. Worst of all, she would be removed from the transplant list if the brain injury proved severe!

Dr. Mulhotra delivered this crushing news in a kind and caring way. We were touched. Sharing this news could not be easy for him. It was then Robin did something that really impressed me. In the midst of her own struggle, she reached out in an effort to comfort the doctor. "You have such a tough job," she said. "We greatly appreciate how caring and compassionate you are. We know sometimes you have to give parents terrible news like this; however, we know it will be OK. God has given us a peace that passes all understanding. We know that no matter what happens everything will be fine."

We returned to Gracyn's room and prayed over her continuously. We prayed for a miracle as we constantly asked her to move her right leg. Soon, we were pretty sure she was moving her right side. It started with an involuntary twitch, but we were sure in time she was moving her right foot on demand.

After some time had passed, a neurosurgeon came by to meet with us. He explained that children's brains have much more plasticity than adults and are much better equipped to heal from brain injuries. He was encouraged by minor movements of Gracyn's right side. He mentioned it seemed she was aware of what was being said to her. This could mean her speech would not be impacted, although we could not be sure until her breathing tube was removed so she could try to talk.

Celebrate Victories

By the next day, everyone was shocked at how well Gracyn was recovering. A second CAT scan confirmed a stroke had occurred. The doctors escalated our hope when they told us the reactions of a patient are much more important indicators than the results of a CAT scan. While, indeed, there had been a stroke, Gracyn was recovering nonetheless.

As we spoke to her of how God was holding her in His powerful arms, Gracyn raised both hands into the air, with her index fingers pointed to her Father in Heaven. Moments later, it was time for the breathing tube to come out. When they removed it, Gracyn immediately tried to talk. However, her throat was full of gunk that needed to be coughed up before her voice could be heard. This was extremely painful and frustrating for her, but Gracyn kept on coughing and fighting. We could tell the pain in her throat was excruciating, yet she desperately wanted to talk. Eventually, with an inaudible whisper, she mouthed the words *I love you* to Robin and me. We could not quite hear it with our ears but our hearts unquestionably felt it. Our eyes filled with tears of joy as we lifted our hands in thanksgiving and praise. God's miracles were raining down on us. We knew our little girl was coming back!

FROM ROBIN'S JOURNAL...

Friday, January 2, 2009

This morning Gracyn started lifting her arms and making fists as if to show she is getting stronger. As Gracyn improves today and can respond verbally more clearly, we will explain to her she will need a new heart to live. She already knows she was very sick, and, indeed, it was her heart. She is well aware of the machine lying on her tummy. But we need to gently inform her of how this will all work. Pray for complete acceptance and understanding. I know the Lord will give her the same peace He has given us. Pray for no depression or worry on her part.

Stop. Stop! Gray just motioned me over and said ever so slowly as she lifted her arms, pointed up, and said, "Jesus, Jesus saved me. I love Him." Then she said, "He can do miracles and I am a miracle."

I am weeping now as I write. I can barely steady my fingers to type. Then she said, "I love you, Daddy, and I love you, Mommy. I love Jesus the most. He is with me every second, and He can do anything."

She put her hands above her head, clasped them, and said, "I'm going to get better because Jesus is doing miracles." (She said this in the sweetest, weakest voice.) Praise You, God Almighty. Wow! Rejoice with us friends.

Throughout the day, we received more positive news: Gracyn's liver and lungs were looking great. After examining her, the kidney specialist said, "I can't explain it, but her kidneys look fine. You aren't going to need me anymore."

Each person who entered her room that day was welcomed by Gracyn's enthusiastic greeting and outstretched arms. She would tell everyone that Jesus was a miracle worker, and she was one of his miracles. One of my close friends commented, "I've never felt closer to God than I did today in Gracyn's hospital room."

REFLECTION:
Believe God still works miracles.

Occasionally, when hearing bad news, I would allow myself to temporarily dwell on feelings of hopelessness. Paralyzing fear would rush in and make me feel like giving up. We had already heard doctors say there was nothing they could do. Gracyn had survived a helicopter transfer that bordered on the impossible. An experimental artificial heart was keeping her alive. Now she was overcoming a stroke that could have ended the entire healing process. It was at times like these when I was extremely grateful for my relationship with God. Because I knew Him, I knew that I could trust Him to ease my fears and remove my feelings of hopelessness. I have seen firsthand God at work in my life, Gracyn's life, my family's lives, and countless other lives. Because of this, I have grown to trust in God and believe that He continues to do the miraculous!

Who among the gods is like you, O LORD? Who is like you— majestic in holiness, awesome in glory, working wonders? (Exod. 15:11)

FROM MY JOURNAL…

Saturday, January 3, 2009

When it was time for her to talk, my little girl told me, in a weak voice with a quivering lip, she loved me. There were no words so sweet to this daddy's ears… especially considering what Gracyn has been through. For a moment I pondered how our Heavenly Father must feel when we lift our weak voices up to Him and proclaim our love for Him.

As the day wore on, we were amazed at the words our daughter would speak. It is vividly clear to us that our little girl had spent some time at the feet of Jesus. The Spirit of the Lord is unquestionably on our sweet child, and so we rejoice! No one would ever choose the road we are walking, but through it all God is using Gracyn to draw her parents, her friends, and others around the world, closer together, closer to God, and closer to eternity.

We understand the road ahead will be full of valleys. The challenge of living in a hospital bed with an artificial heart attached while waiting for a new heart undoubtedly will be difficult to fathom for a nine-year-old. Yet, today we celebrate. Today we stand on the mountaintop and lift our eyes unto the One who is able to provide more than we could ever hope or imagine. Today and every day, regardless of circumstance, we will praise Jesus, "the miracle worker," who holds us close in His healing arms.

Miracles are God's power at work. Even though He's a good and caring God, I have found God only performs miracles as they line up with His perfect will…and in His precise timing, not on demand or when we think we need it. Though we should not be shy about making our specific requests known to the Lord, we should open ourselves to accept His will no matter what that may be.

As Robin and I prayed or asked others to pray, we only wanted a miracle that would be within God's will and align with His plan for our lives. True faith is not trusting God will do what we want Him to do, but trusting what He does is what we need exactly when we need it.

[Jesus] withdrew about a stone's throw beyond them, knelt down and prayed, "Father, if you are willing, take this cup from me; yet not my will, but yours be done." (Luke 22:41-42)

From Gracyn's Heart…

When I started waking up from my surgery, it was really weird because people looked very blurry to me. They seemed like they had more than one head and moved around like robots. I could hear them making noise, but I couldn't understand what they were saying to me. It seemed like a weird dream.

I knew I was going to be OK because when I was asleep Jesus had let me know I was going to get better. He let me know He would do miracles and that I was a miracle. It is hard to explain because it wasn't like He had talked to me with a voice. It was just like He made me feel these things inside. It is so hard to explain in words. All I can say is I had the most deep, holy, and pure feeling that God was with me and taking care of me the whole time.

As the medicine wore off, I remember hearing music and this ticking sound that was off-key and off-beat. At first I thought it was coming from the CD-player, but then I realized it was coming from a big box beside me. There was a swooshing noise down by my stomach. Later I found out this was the Berlin Heart®.

My mom explained it to me first. I really didn't like it very much. However, the more I heard about it, I loved it. It was one of God's miracles He had promised. It was a miracle machine that kept me alive.

CHAPTER 6

WHEN YOU DON'T THINK YOU CAN DO IT

WITH THE MIRACLE OF the Berlin Heart® surgery behind us, we began a new phase of our journey, which resembled a rollercoaster ride with its dramatic ups and downs and unpredictable turns. New challenges and unexpected crises were sandwiched between periods of sheer boredom and drops in morale. While Gracyn struggled mightily throughout the journey, she faithfully took it all in stride. We have always known Gracyn as an extremely resolute child, but we had no idea how fiercely determined our little girl could be.

LEARNING TO LIVE DAY-TO-DAY

We learned to approach each day by faith. Celebrating the mountain tops and confidently trusting God to carry us through the valleys, we would tackle one problem at a time as we faced each new challenge.

Some of the best advice we received came from Dr. Nykanen back on Christmas morning. He had advised us to mentally envision a positive, long-range outcome while focusing all our energies and attention to each 24-hour period before us. In essence, this is what a walk of faith is all about: trusting the eventual outcome to God while continually seeking enough strength and provision from Him for each new day.

We had no idea as to the intensity or the duration of the battle we would face. Over the next months, we would experience sorrow and elation, terror and peace, extreme doubt and firm faith, our utter weakness and God's limitless strength. The mental, physical, emotional, and spiritual battles were constant. Doing whatever we could to get by, we truly were living life day-to-day as survivors.

FROM ROBIN'S JOURNAL...

Tuesday, January 6, 2009

Gracyn is recovering so beautifully; however, it truly is an emotional/physical rollercoaster. We're trying to help Gray understand this. Finally, last night, we saw her cry. The first thing I, as a mom, wanted to do was scoop up my child into my arms and comfort her. I can't do this as I can only get as close as the bedrail allows. I can't wait to just hold Gray. I miss that so much.

Poor Gracyn shared her thoughts with us: "I just want to go home. I just want to get out of here and go home."

We held her hands, stroked her face, and told her it's completely OK to feel this way. It's very normal to have these emotions. When you wake up in a hospital (many times during the night) and it's a new day, it all sort of hits you once again. Oh, my goodness, I'm still here. Am I ever leaving?

For the first time, I heard her ask, "When am I leaving?" And I could only tell her, "Exactly when God wants you to. He'll bring your heart at the perfect time."

I then explained the peace the Lord has given Kris and me about this. She listened intently and wanted to possess this peace. So we prayed together once again. "Lord, give us the strength to make it through another day and grant us the peace of knowing you are in control. Continue to move each mountain along the way and carry us in Your loving arms."

Learning to Handle On-going Struggles

There were struggles we would face on an ever-occurring basis that would sometimes bring Gracyn to the brink of saying, "I can't do this anymore." These battles were heart-wrenching. While our efforts often appeared to be futile, we had no choice but to keep pressing on, no matter how senseless it might seem.

1. Handling the Struggle with Eating

Gracyn initially received nutrients through a feeding tube. Once this tube was removed, it was a constant struggle to get her to eat. When she did not feel well, the last thing she wanted was constant probing to eat more…of anything. Yet, we needed to make sure she got enough calories to gain weight and sustain her health.

Robin and I tried to stuff Gracyn with high-calorie protein shakes and ice cream, anything we could get her to ingest. Hoping and praying we could coax her to eat more, we often got take-out food from one of her favorite restaurants.

We never thought we would pray so often and fervently for one of our children to eat more.

2. Handling the Struggle with Nausea and Pain

After being so sick, having tubes inserted into the top of her belly, and experiencing constant pain, it is not surprising Gracyn suffered with a lot of nausea. Rarely was there a day she did not have a stomach ache, queasiness, or a case of vomiting.

Though she modeled steely determination, Gracyn struggled daily with pain. Her arms turned purple from the bruising of constant blood-thinning shots. Physical, occupational, and respiratory therapy required Gracyn to fight through the pain. Regular dressing changes and necessary testing procedures were excruciating for her to endure and frustrating for us to watch.

From Robin's journal…

Friday, February 6, 2009
I just watched my daughter scream out in pain
over and over as her sweet nurse tried to remove

sticky tape and adjust a PICC line in her arm for the THIRD time tonight. (It's now 11:36 p.m. She stared into my eyes, crying out for help, "Mommy, Mommy!!!") It seemed like an eternity.

I don't even know how to describe the anguish I, as a mom, have watching my little girl suffer in pain. I stepped around the corner after she was calmed down and LOST IT!

How did You feel, God, the night Your Son cried out from the cross?" I asked. "Oh, Father, You know how I felt just now. God, I can't wait for the day when You heal this daughter of Yours and she walks from here proclaiming Your greatness forevermore. I know it's coming. Thank You in advance for what You are going to do."

3. HANDLING THE STRUGGLE WITH MEDICATIONS

Four times each day (including 4:00 a.m.) Gracyn would have to take her many medicines. There were medications for her blood, heart, and stomach; to increase her appetite; to reduce nausea. There were medicines to offset medicines. We were never in short supply of medicine!

Gracyn had never swallowed a pill in her life. Initially, we tried all the tricks. We ground the pills up and put them in applesauce, grape juice, smoothies…anything to get them down. Getting her to swallow her meds was one of our most painful and long-standing battles.

Sometimes forcefully, often with tears, the medicine would have to go down one way or another. Many times she would vomit it right back up. Then she would have to take the medication over again.

Eventually, we had no choice. We empathized with Gracyn's situation, but it was time for some "tough love." One night we demanded Gracyn learn to swallow pills. Despite our sympathy for her, we had no choice but to relentlessly stick with it. After numerous "I can'ts," many prayers, continuous tears, countless pleadings, and, ultimately, stern commands, Gracyn learned to swallow pills.

After all she had been through, it was amazing how difficult this fear of swallowing pills was for her to overcome. Yet, with God's help, she did it. While this did not stop the nausea or the frequent vomiting, it did make taking the medicine easier, less time-consuming, and much less stressful on all of us.

4. HANDLING THE STRUGGLE WITH INFECTIONS

Keeping a potential transplant patient free from infection is a daunting task. Due to her condition and long-term hospitalization, Gracyn was highly susceptible. Keeping her free from infection was critical. Should a donor heart come available at a time when she had an infection, they would have to pass on the heart and prolong the wait. Unfortunately, over the months of her stay at Shands, Gracyn contracted numerous infections. Each time she did, treatment required powerful antibiotic drugs, which would make her more nauseous than ever and limit her physical activity.

One morning Gracyn developed a high fever. To counter it, they once again administered strong antibiotics. As I walked her over to brush her teeth, she began feeling really cold. She went ahead and took her normal morning medicines and then began shivering uncontrollably.

I carried her to bed and covered her with warm blankets as she grew increasingly agitated and began to cry out. The fear in her eyes startled me. Gracyn became frantic as her oxygenation numbers dropped rapidly. Her nurse hit the emergency call button and the terrifying sound of the distress alarm pierced through the PICU. Her room quickly filled with doctors and nurses. Gracyn, Robin, and I experienced terrifying flashbacks to that night in Orlando when Gracyn thought she was going to die. We had no idea what was going on. Once again, it seemed we were staring death in the face. *Not again! Not this hopeless feeling! Please God!* Our emotions were running wild. All we could do was pray, trust in God, and watch helplessly as medical professionals surrounded our little girl.

Eventually, the medical staff was convinced she had "gone septic." Apparently bacteria had entered her body through her PICC line—a central line used to administer medications directly to her blood stream. These bacteria had showered her body and caused it to go into shock.

This condition is critical for any patient. However, it produced tremendous anxiety in Gracyn's case. The team had not before experienced a septic shower with a Berlin Heart® patient. There were some extremely tense moments.

Eventually her condition improved. Within an hour Gracyn was smiling, telling us she loves us, and thanking God and her doctors for helping her through this most frightening ordeal.

5. Handling the Struggle with Seizures

Infections were not the only low points in Gracyn's recovery. One morning Gracyn felt as though she had peanut butter in her mouth and could not get it out. While lying in bed her face started twitching. It wasn't a major movement, but she was unable to control the twitch. When her nurse saw what was happening, she called for immediate help. Gracyn was suffering from a seizure.

Quickly administering anti-seizure medications, the medical staff immediately took Gracyn for a CAT scan. That test showed what looked like bleeding around her brain. This was a major concern because they had continually thinned her blood so the Berlin pumps could run efficiently. However, thin blood is extremely dangerous if the brain is bleeding.

Over the next two days she endured so much. Four CAT scans. Countless neurological exams. Additional medications which caused the nausea to worsen. Steady visits from eye doctors, neurologists, infectious disease specialists, and brain surgeons. The last straw was having her eyes dilated to see behind them, to which Gracyn cried out, "I just want to be left alone."

After two days of what seemed like torture, she finally wanted to know why she was not allowed to eat anything. Robin cautiously explained she could not eat because if they determined her brain was bleeding, they might have to do some surgery to relieve the pressure. With a dropped jaw and a look of total bewilderment, Gracyn blurted out, "What?! So now I need a heart transplant and brain surgery? Before this all I ever used to worry about was bee stings and mosquito bites!"

Her blunt exclamation caused us to burst out in uncontrollable laughter. It was good to laugh again. It was a great release of all that was terrifying us.

Eventually, they ruled out most of the major concerns. Gracyn was allowed to return to "normal" hospital life, including eating again. However, they kept Gray on anti-seizure medications for months to follow.

Fighting all of these physical battles while attached to a machine 24/7 and living in the confines of a small hospital room often caused our weakened child to think she could not take it any longer. Children should not have to face such difficulties. It definitely wasn't fair! Robin and I, too, would often wonder how much more she could endure. Ever-occurring challenges would make us feel, at times, like giving up. By learning to depend wholly on God's strength to carry us through, we were able to handle all these struggles, overcome the sense of unfairness, and keep moving ahead.

FROM MY JOURNAL...

Sunday, February 8, 2009

It's the dawn of a new week. Despite the promise the Son brings to us, we are growing weary. The weight of this journey is taxing. The pain, anxiety, and

sorrow that assault our daughter greatly trouble our
hearts.

At times we cry out to God and implore Him to
spare us this pain: "Oh, God, don't desert us. Don't be
far from us. Lord, hear our prayer. Listen to our cry
for help. Savior, come quickly to heal this infirmity."

The burden overwhelms us until we remember the
weight of this worry is not ours to carry. Indeed, this
battle is the Lord's and not our own. He has a perfect
plan in which He conducts all things. This plan promises
hope and a future, but never does it guarantee an easy
road. So we wait expectantly for His will to play out.

"Father, You have lifted Gracyn from the pit of
death. You are creating and orchestrating a new song
for her to sing. It is a song that draws others to Your
glory, a song of praise that inspires others to worship
and proclaim their trust in You. As we focus on You, our
own load lightens, and we find great joy in the good
works You are doing. So we thank You for placing us in
the front row to experience so many of Your miracles.
And we press on confidently in faith knowing You will
carry us through this storm."

REFLECTION:
Rely on God's perfect strength.

We could not have survived this long ordeal without God's supernatural strength in our lives. It would have been unbearable. All the ups and downs would have torn us apart. Often, when we felt completely drained and at the point of giving up, we would cry out to God for just enough strength for that next step. We've found His strength is perfect when our strength is gone. When we are weak, He is strong.

> But he said to me, "My grace is sufficient for you, for power is made perfect in weakness." So, I will boast all the more gladly of my weaknesses, so that the power of Christ may dwell in me. Therefore I am content in weaknesses, insults, hardships, persecutions, and calamities for the sake of Christ; for whenever I am weak, then I am strong. (2 Cor. 12:9-10 nrsv)

I cannot imagine surviving any of this without God to lean on. We received the very best medical care and support available, yet we needed more help—a different kind of help—to handle all the struggles. Apart from God, we would have been too weak. The heartache and stress would have been too much. In Him we received the strength necessary for us to face any hardship and the power to overcome each challenge that came our way.

> Do you not know? Have you not heard? The LORD is the everlasting God, the Creator of the ends of the earth. He will not grow tired or weary, and his understanding no one can fathom. He gives strength to the weary and increases the power of the weak. (Isa. 40:28-29)

FROM GRACYN'S HEART...

Each morning when I woke up, I would always pray that nothing bad would happen that day. It seemed like whenever bad things would happen, it would always become so difficult to handle. A lot of days I would wake up with a stomach ache. I knew I had to eat and take medicine. However, because of my stomach ache, I didn't want to. Then, when I had to do it, I would usually throw up. It was so hard.

My mom and dad were always there for me. I wanted to make them proud while I was in the hospital. Taking medicine, which I had to take lots of, always freaked me out. The medicine tasted awful. It made me feel sick, like I was going to gag. My parents were always really nice to me in the hospital, but one night they got very harsh with me about swallowing pills. I didn't think I could do it, but they forced me into it. We prayed a lot. Then, when I finally swallowed one, I just laughed because it was so easy. All I had to do was put one on my tongue and take a sip of water. I take them so easily now!

So many bad things happened—like throwing up, having a seizure, bandage changes that hurt, and other things. When it got really bad, I just wanted to scream. I always would wish it were just a dream. But no matter how tough it got, I would pray for strength to make it through and patience to wait for a heart so I could go home. No matter what I faced, I knew I could pray and that God would give me peace, comfort, and the power to make it through.

PART THREE

FACING THE LONG HAUL

*For video, pictures, and interviews that relate
to Part Three, go to www.gracyn.org.*

Chapter 7

WHEN YOU ARE
SICK OF WAITING

WHEN WE FIND OURSELVES waiting for a big event, we might know how long our wait will be. When we get anxious for Christmas, birthdays, or summer vacation to roll around, we know the big date. That wasn't the case while waiting for Gray's heart transplant. There was no way anyone could tell us when a heart would come available.

If only there had been a date to shoot for or some sort of target to motivate her, our family could have marked off the days on a calendar or had a countdown for Gracyn. Waiting without knowing became torturous. Hours clicked slowly into days, days turned into weeks, and weeks passed into months. Christmas, New Year's, Valentine's Day, Easter all rolled around, and we found ourselves waiting.

WAITING IS THE HARDEST PART

Of all the struggles and pains Gracyn endured, what was the greatest source of despair? Her not knowing when this ordeal would conclude. We would have loved to ease her sorrow by telling her when.

Gracyn would say through tears, "You always tell me I will be home someday. I just want to know when that someday is!"

We wore out the phrase, "You will get your heart in God's perfect timing."

As much as we believed that statement to be true, the more time passed, the tougher it became to stay focused and positive. For Gracyn, waiting truly was the hardest part.

FROM ROBIN'S JOURNAL...

Tuesday, January 20, 2009

Kris and I sat silently today as Gracyn cried out in despair over her desire to return home. She is growing increasingly tired of waiting. As I held my little girl in the corner chair by the window, I felt sickened by my inability to comfort her. Her requests are simple: to get herself up to go to the bathroom, to not need a nurse to reach something at the end of her bed, to run outside and play with her dog, to do her homework at her special spot at the kitchen island, to sing karaoke upstairs in the playroom.

My eyes welled with tears as hers became red and swollen from crying. When she reached the end, I quietly whispered in her ear, "Daddy and I would trade places with you in an instant. We wish it were us and not you. We would love to carry this burden for you."

Her moans quieted as she listened, and then I said, "Daddy and I can't do that, but you know who can?

Jesus! Jesus will carry this burden, sweet baby girl. Jesus died on the cross for such a time as this. He's standing ready to carry it all for you, for me, for Daddy, for each and every one of us. All we have to do is hand it over to Him. He'll carry you through. He has a plan, and His timing is perfect!"

This is a hard lesson to learn. If it's hard for me as an adult, how much harder is it for my nine-year-old daughter, trapped in a hospital room with a machine attached to her body? I can truly say I've learned this lesson the hard way. I'm glad to know the freedom that lies within His promises. I'm ashamed it took my daughter almost losing her life for me to "get it." I wait and rest, safe and secure in His arms. Seems I still have more to learn and more to hand over to Him. It's a daily battle, but a battle He will win.

Walking the halls of the PICU at Shands, we became aware of so many heart-wrenching stories. Daily we encountered the parents of kids of all ages, with different challenges and varying prognoses, but all waiting for something. Some of the parents were somber and quiet. Others would talk about their challenges and struggles. We shared a special bond with them. Like us, they dealt with fear, suffering, and sorrow. Like us, they were waiting.

FROM ROBIN'S JOURNAL...

Wednesday, March 25, 2009

I am looking over at Gracyn as she sleeps so soundly. What a beautiful, little girl. I treasure every minute, every special moment we've shared since being here.

Sometimes when I walk down the halls of the PICU, I feel like I'm living in a dream. I hear babies crying and children moaning. I've seen rooms stripped bare overnight because a patient has passed away. I've seen and heard things I never knew existed.

I've watched our precious angel suffer over and over. I haven't been with our boys for more than a couple nights in a row in three months. I can't put into words how much I miss them. I tell you this, I HATE IT!!! I can't stand it. I don't understand any of it, but I am comforted by a tender, loving, caring, giving, merciful, omniscient, omnipotent, faithful God. How must He feel watching all this?

"Lord, I'll hang on with You. I'll hang on to You. I'm waiting! Carry me, Father. I am tired and weary. But, I am still and know You are God. I love You, Lord."

FINDING JOY IS THE KEY IN WAITING

As we waited and waited...and then waited some more, we did our best to entertain ourselves. It got so monotonous that Gracyn invented her own word to describe her days: "totalboringness."

Each day we tried to overcome totalboringness. We made up ridiculous characters that I would act out to break the monotony. These included the worst nurse in the world, Nurse Hearse, (think about that one for a moment); the world's strangest doctor, Dr. Doofball; the world's strictest school teacher, Yoy Swabstick; a constipated bunny rabbit; and many other wild characters. Gracyn called these characters "dumbiots," which I think is the combination of *dumb* and *idiot*, but I'm not really sure. When you spend as much time as we did in a hospital, you come up with some pretty crazy things to humor yourself.

From Gracyn's journal…

Friday, March 6, 2009

It was a pretty good day again for me. It started with my dad making eggs. He needs some serious cooking lessons. Last time they were bland, and this time they were all soggy, drenched, and gooey. I only ate one bite. Mom needs to teach him how to cook eggs, I think. I did really good at school. I did reading, writing, and English today.

My dad likes to act like this really goofy teacher who tries to be strict and calls me Sweet Tea. It's pretty crazy but fun. I wrote a story about finding a money tree, and it made my dad laugh. It was pretty funny, I guess. We had a lot of fun today acting like dumbiots.

Tonight my dad went over to the apartment and grilled me my favorite steak. My protein is low, so I have to eat steak a lot. That's kind of good because steak is my favorite. My dad makes steak way better than he makes eggs. I guess Mom should make the eggs and Dad will make the steak.

I guess I should take my medicine now and get ready for bed. Thanks for praying for me. I really want to go home, but I know God is in control of His plan for me. Goodnight, Gracyn

Watching videos on our laptop became a favorite pastime. Did you know there were nine seasons of the show *Little House on the Prairie*? There are around twenty episodes per season. Do the math as to how many of those episodes we watched. After watching a couple back-to-back episodes, I heard Gracyn tell Robin in amazement, "Dad's phone rang like five times, and he didn't even answer it!"

I was humbled. I had no idea how much our sharing this time together meant to her. It is a shame it took something drastic like this for me to understand how important it is to spend time alone with my daughter, fully devoted to something she wants to do. In the past I was always too busy with work, preoccupied with something else, or too interested in other things to give her my full attention. I am so thankful for the father-daughter time we shared that literally changed my heart while we waited for God to provide her with a new heart.

FROM MY JOURNAL...

Friday, March 27, 2009

Gracyn and I are snuggled close to each other watching another of her beloved *Little House on the Prairie* episodes. As she dozes off to sleep for the night, I am overcome with thankfulness for the opportunities to spend this time with my beloved daughter.

I can't explain the pain a father feels watching his daughter endure so much. It has been three months since Gracyn was airlifted to the intensive care unit here at Shands. As I glance at her arms, I see countless bruises from the shots administered to thin her blood. Of course, you can't miss the tubes embedded in her body that provide the lifeline from the artificial heart to her arteries.

It really is overwhelming to realize that only three months ago she was fully healthy. And now I find myself wondering how much more she can endure. Will it ever end?

As the pain of fatherhood reaches the depths of my soul, there is peace in knowing my Father in Heaven understands this pain. I am comforted by the reminder He watched His Son endure much more so that I might call Him Savior. Isn't it reassuring to call upon a God who knows our pain and has a plan to overcome it?

"Lord, teach me to view this from Your perspective. I know You have a perfect plan. I trust You will reveal it clearly. So Lord, I wait.

I wait in faith...acknowledging You are in control.
I wait in confidence...knowing You are almighty.
I wait with expectancy...knowing Your plan is perfect.
I wait in thankfulness...for what You are going to do.
I wait in dependence...knowing You are all I need.
And I wait in stillness...knowing You are my God."

REFLECTION: RECOGNIZE GOD'S PLAN IS WORTH THE WAIT.

Although it often comes wrapped in difficulty, waiting can be a gift. As we worked our way through the challenges and tried to patiently wait on the Lord, the gift began to reveal itself. For our family, the gift of waiting produced faith, hope, and love in our lives. It brought us together in unity and strengthened us for the long haul. We grew closer as a family, to friends, and in our relationship with our God. God absolutely had a plan for allowing our family to wait for Gracyn's healing.

> *"For I know the plans I have for you," declares the LORD, "plans to prosper you and not to harm you, plans to give you hope and a future." (Jer. 29:11)*

From my journal…

Friday, April 3, 2009

Sure this journey is long and painful. We keep wondering when it will ever end. I long to just wipe away my daughter's suffering. I would give everything just to take her home with me. I would trade places with her in a heartbeat. Yet, we all know I can't do that. All I can do is wait with her, encourage her, and keep trusting in God and His plan. Her healing is totally out of our hands and fully in His.

As we continue waiting, I'm beginning to see this valley for what it truly is: a vale not strictly of pain but of true blessing. After all, how many dads do you know who get to spend this much time with their daughters? Had it not been for this journey, I would have surely missed knowing her so intimately. At the base of this gorge, I've discovered what it really means to be a father. I've learned much about love. For the first time, I understand how to fully yield my hopes, dreams, and ambitions to the One who already holds them all. You see this is not my valley I'm passing through but His.

"I thank You, Lord, for the valleys, for the fruit that grows there, and especially for the blessings of faith, hope, and love that inspire mountains to move in Your name and for Your glory."

The LORD is my shepherd…he restores my soul. He guides me in the paths of righteousness for his name's sake. Even though I walk through the valley of the shadow of death, I will fear no evil, for you are with me. (Ps. 23:1a, 3-4)

While our family waited on God to act, He waited patiently on us to receive the many good benefits of waiting. We have come to appreciate the wait, to thank God for the wait. Although we pray we don't ever go through this "totalboringness" again!

I am still confident of this: I will see the goodness of the LORD in the land of the living. Wait for the LORD; be strong and take heart and wait for the LORD. (Ps. 27:13-14)

From Gracyn's Heart…

I would always get really sad when I started wondering if I was ever going to get out of the hospital. When I would ask my parents when I could go home, they would always say, "Soon." Then, when it was taking a really long time, they started telling me they didn't know when, but that I would get a heart and go home in God's perfect timing. I believed that. Still it was so hard. I was so tired of waiting.

Waiting in a hospital is no fun. You can't do all the things you want to do. When you are waiting for a heart transplant, it's really hard and scary. You want that day to come so you can go home, but you are worried and frightened because it means you will have to have surgery again.

You have to do your best to have fun and come up with things to do when you are stuck in the hospital. Acting like dumbiots was totally weird and very strange, but we had to do something to raise the level of fun-ness.

Waiting brought me closer to God because I prayed so much. It also brought me closer to my parents because they were with me all the time. Normally—when I am busy—I don't stop and pray like I need to. In the hospital, I would pray way more than before I got sick. Probably the best thing about waiting is spending more time praying with God.

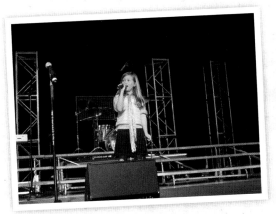

Gracyn singing in her school chapel service
1 month prior to her illness

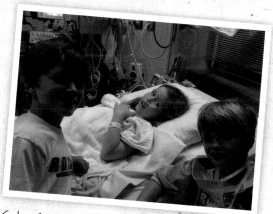

Cole, Gracyn, Brooks at Arnold Palmer
Hospital, Christmas Eve, 2008

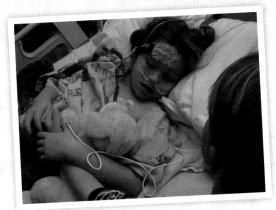

Gracyn holds Brooks' hand while coming to
from Berlin Heart® surgery

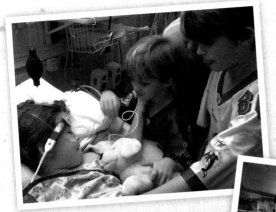

Saying hi to Gracyn as she wakes from coma

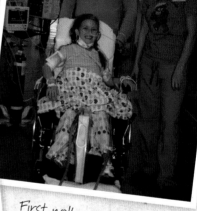

First walk around Shands Hospital PICU with Dad and nurse Stephanie

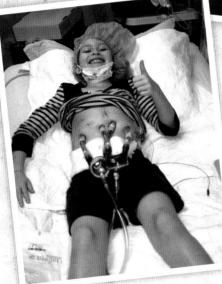

A view of the Berlin Heart® pumps during one of Gray's bandage changes

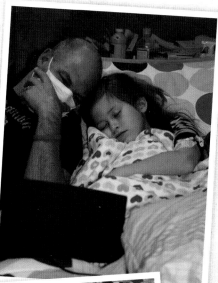

Watching another "Little House on the Prairie" episode

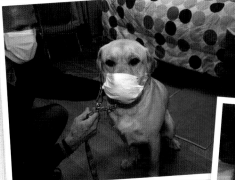

Dr. Biscuit making his rounds

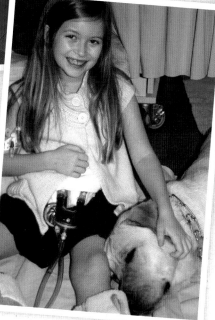

Gracyn and Biscuit hanging out in her hospital room

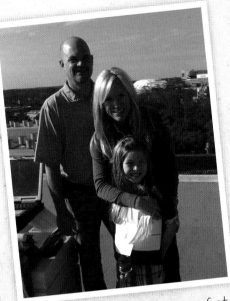

Getting some sunshine on the roof at
Shands Hospital

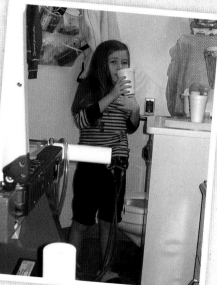

Hospital life got much easier when
Gracyn learned to swallow pills

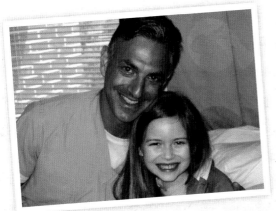

Our surgeon, Dr. Mark Bleiweis,
aka "Wise Eyes"

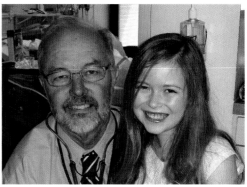

Gracyn's cardiologist at Shands Hospital,
Dr. Jay Fricker

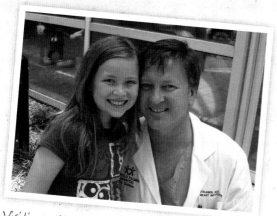

Visiting with Dr. David Nykanen at
Arnold Palmer Hospital

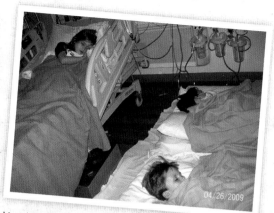

Hospital slumber party

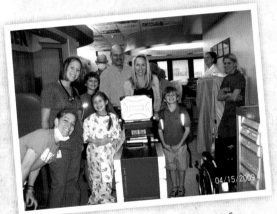

Heading down to the operating room for
Gracyn's heart transplant

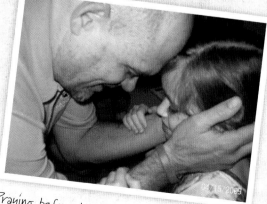

Praying before heart transplant surgery

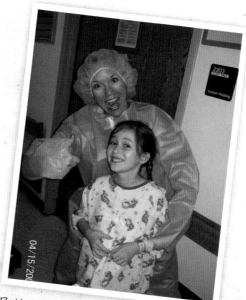

Robin and Gracyn before entering
O.R. doors on April 15, 2009

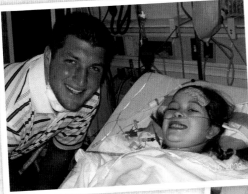

Florida Gator QB Tim Tebow
visits the day after Gracyn's
transplant

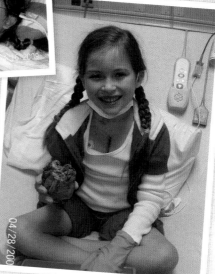

Gracyn holds her own heart in her
hand

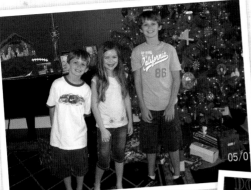

Christmas Day finally celebrated
at our home in May

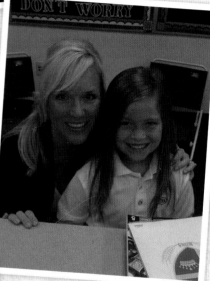

Gracyn returns to school for
the first day of fifth grade

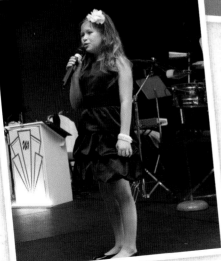

Gracyn sings at the annual heart ball
of the American Heart Association

CHAPTER
8

WHEN YOU JUST WANT
TO BE NORMAL AGAIN

THERE WAS NOTHING NORMAL about waking up each morning, month after month, in a hospital room. Though many of the days were similar and routines had become common place, it never felt normal. Hospital life was far removed from our normal family life at home in Orlando.

Some of the simplest things had become quite a production—anything but normal—as Gracyn learned about living in a PICU while being sustained by a Berlin Heart®. She made many friends and was treated so well by the team at Shands. Gracyn, however, would have given anything to be normal again and able to return home.

FROM MY JOURNAL...

Sunday, January 11, 2009

We were thrilled today as Gracyn walked down the hall of the PICU and then back to her room. This process takes a nurse moving the medicine cart and tube drain pan, another nurse pushing the Berlin Heart® power unit, a physical therapist supporting Gracyn while she walks, and an excited mom and dad cheering her along the way.

Physically, Gracyn continues to make great progress, but, mentally, she is struggling. She is not talking or smiling nearly as much as a few days ago. She seems much more sad and frustrated with her situation. It is tough not knowing when she will be able to get a new heart and go home. Honestly, it's getting mentally tough on all of us.

Unless you've experienced it, you cannot comprehend the anguish of seeing your little one cry in pain from bandage changes or an accidental bump of a drain tube, or hearing her softly whimper, "I just want to go home." The fact is we all just want to go home. Our seven-year-old, Brooks, broke down in Robin's arms last night with that same request. Cole says he can't wait until we move back into our house and live like a normal family again.

SEPARATION FROM HOME AND FAMILY

One of our most difficult challenges throughout this ordeal was dealing with the separation of our family. Robin and I had rented a small apartment less than a mile from Shands so we could be close to Gracyn. For the first couple of months, we both stayed in Gainesville full-time while our boys stayed at their grandparents' home in

Orlando, one hundred miles away. While we were so blessed to have my parents and close friends who were able to care for our boys in our absence, it was still a major struggle. We all longed for our family to be back together and resume a life as normal as possible.

From Robin's journal...

Monday, January 12, 2009

We didn't see many smiles from Gracyn today. We heard, through tears, how she wants to go home and sit in her normal spot at the kitchen island, sleep in her bed, sing on her stage in the playroom, lay on the sofa in the family room. It breaks my heart. She held me close tonight when I lifted her back to bed. She whispered in my ear, "Don't leave. I love it when you're here, Mommy." I rested my head on her shoulder and, through my mask, kissed her like a momma does. I got as close as I possibly could (while balancing on one knee, being careful not to hurt her) and loved on her.

As hard as it is to leave, we did. When Kris and I got in the car, I shared my heart about our boys. I miss them terribly. It's killing me not to have our family together. I spoke of our youngest son, Brooks (7), and my concerns for both the boys being separated from us for this long. Just then I pulled up an email from our 11-year-old son, Cole. I started reading and began weeping. Kris took my phone and read it as I sat in the passenger seat, sobbing. I couldn't control myself. Here is what my son sent me...

Hi Mom, it's Cole. I love you so much! I am trying my best to get my homework done and make you pleased. I know that what's going on is hard for you as the mother and all, but this is also very hard for me too. I miss your gentle voice in the morning waking me up, the delicious smell of your homemade scrambled eggs, and the "Good Morning" song you sing to us. Sometimes during school, I find myself daydreaming about you coming to pick me up and taking me to Gainesville with you and Dad and spending quality time with my precious family. Over the last couple weeks, I have been so touched by my sister's preachings. She's making me realize that God is the only one who can heal her and make her feel better. She is truly in God's mighty arms. Momma, it could take a while, but I don't care as long as my sister comes home safe and sound. I just finished writing a letter to Gracyn, and I felt led to write one to you. Well, Mom, the point of this letter is to let you know that I'm praying and love you guys so much. I'm getting a little teary-eyed as I write this, but it doesn't matter because I love you and always will. Momma, have a great night. I hope you really like this letter. You are my role model and hero. I LOVE YOU!!

As I look at it again, I become emotional. I can't describe what this feels like: one child clinging to life

with the help of a miraculous machine and two sweet
boys trying to go on as if everything is fine. Ouch!
Many have asked how I'm holding up. Well, today has
been rough. I'm tired and weary from tending to Gray
and terribly missing my boys.

Gracyn missed her brothers. She loved it when they would come
to the hospital and visit her most every weekend. We did our best
to manufacture our "normal lifestyle" while living in the PICU.
We had family dinners seated by the nursing stations. We hung a
Nerf basketball hoop in one of the hallways where our boys played
out countless fantasy games. Nurses, other staff, and doctors would
sometimes join in the fun. On a few occasions we even brought
Gracyn's beloved yellow lab, Biscuit, in for visits. We had a Super
Bowl party, brought in a chocolate fountain for Valentine's Day, and
held an Easter egg hunt on our floor as we strived for some semblance
of normalcy. Despite all these efforts, normalcy was nowhere to be
found.

New Appreciation for Life

Surviving all the turmoil associated with Gracyn's medical crisis
provided us with a new appreciation for the gift of life—normal or
not. We enjoyed the simplest of "normal" family interaction and
time shared together with greater appreciation.

While it's really hard to imagine spending such a large amount
of time in a hospital—especially with active, energetic, and adven-
turous boys visiting regularly—we loved being together so much

that we just made it happen. As weekends would conclude, saying goodbye to our boys became one of the toughest things we would face. It was hardest on Gracyn because she always wanted to go with them back to Orlando…back to her normal life.

One weekend we decided to let the boys stay an extra day so we could enjoy a bit more time together. It was a beautiful day outside and a "normal" routine day for us, or so it seemed…

FROM ROBIN'S JOURNAL…

Monday, March 2, 2009

Have you ever been really scared? Well, we were today! The first part of the day was quite normal for us in the PICU. Picture our boys sliding around the halls on rolling chairs, shooting Nerf rockets at random targets, and creating games with anything that vaguely resembles a ball. Picture me trying to corral them long enough to go over schoolwork for a few minutes. Gray hung out, watched the madness, and periodically joined in.

By 2:00 p.m. we all needed a break. We inquired about a trip to the roof. Joy, a respiratory therapist and a member of the helicopter life flight team, volunteered to take us up to the helicopter pad for a look around. After clearing it with "the big cheese," Dr. Wise Eyes, we grabbed our coats and off we went. As Gracyn's machine has a battery life of only thirty minutes, we planned to go up to the roof, hang out for

about ten minutes and come right back...all in time to
plug-in and recharge. No problem.

We made it to the roof and enjoyed some fresh air
for a bit. It was a beautiful day—clear and crisp. Our
whole family was glad to escape the PICU, if only for
a time. The Berlin alarm sounded at twenty minutes to
remind us we had ten minutes until we needed to plug
in and recharge the battery. We began our trek back
to the room: down the ramp and into the elevator.

Making a strange sound when its doors closed, the
elevator stalled. At first, I thought I must be imagining
things, but reality quickly clicked in. WE WERE
STUCK IN THE ELEVATOR, AND THE BERLIN
BATTERY HAD LESS THAN TEN MINUTES
CHARGE REMAINING!

All adults kept their cool for the sake of the kids.
Very calmly, Joy called on her cell phone for help.
After that we waited. Eventually the thirty-minute
alarm sounded on the Berlin, and I silenced it. Gracyn
was fine. She never flinched or showed any sign of
worry. After the thirty-minute alarm sounded, an alarm
went off every minute. This was starting to make me
sweat, but I knew God had it all under control. We
knew He hadn't brought us this far just to let it all
end in an elevator stuck between floors. We did not
panic and, thankfully, the Berlin battery never fully
discharged.

Eventually the problem was resolved, and the door opened! We raced off the elevator and into the PICU. We weren't expecting the group of very concerned doctors—especially Dr. Bleiweis—and nurses, who had heard what was going on and awaiting our arrival. This was all super serious. Praise God, He had it all worked out for us. What are the odds of our getting trapped in an elevator?!

It's amazing how something as dramatic and implausible as our elevator scare can slow life down and allow us to see things more clearly. As time became more critical and we more helpless to do anything about it, I was profoundly reminded of the value of every second of life that God has given us. This incident was a stark reminder—as if we needed one—of the seriousness in relying on an artificial heart to stay alive. Even simple things like spending ten minutes on a rooftop enjoying a beautiful day could have devastating consequences if something went wrong. As much as we desired to make things more normal, we needed to accept our situation, wait patiently on God, and continue to place our focus on trusting Him. He would determine our new normal in His way and in His perfect timing.

REFLECTION:
FOCUS ON WHAT'S MOST IMPORTANT.

Later, reflecting on the elevator scare, I knew what had transpired there was for a reason. This became a common theme through Gracyn's illness: God using situations which were far from normal to teach me what truly is most important in my normal life.

From my journal…

Monday, January 19, 2009

There is a lesson God is revealing through my kids that I'd like to share with you. When Gracyn gets frustrated or saddened about her situation, she always proclaims she just wants to be normal again. She wants to be in her normal room and play with her normal friends. She longs for her normal life back. Interestingly, my boys are crying out for the exact same thing: normalcy. They just want us all together again in the same place and to return to our normal life together.

I have to admit, I've spent most my life striving not to be normal. Those who know me well can attest to that! Now, don't get me wrong. I am not advocating complacency in any way. I fully believe God wants us to grow every day, to step out and make a difference and allow Him to do totally abnormal things through us.

Yet, tonight I realize what a blessing our normal life can be. With that in mind, I am thanking God for my normal life. I thank Him that my kids want their normal life back as well. I am beginning to understand how God does incredible things through ordinary people who are grateful and content in their normal everyday surroundings. While it's great to go out and courageously be all we can be, we should not take the normal for granted. We should learn to appreciate every day and remember what matters most.

I began to understand there was a big disconnect between what I thought my priorities were and what my actions in my normal life proved them to be. My actions revealed what my "normal" really was: a life lived with too little attention to the most important relationships in my life—God, my family, and my friends—and too much focus on my work and my own accomplishments.

Before Gracyn's illness, I loved God and my family, but I don't think I had my priorities properly in order. Most of my time was spend focusing on my work, providing for my family, and trying to serve the Lord. I was a CEO, had done quite well professionally, and had written a book about serving God in the workplace. Yet, in the elevator that day, none of those major accomplishments seemed to matter much. While trapped and fearing for Gracyn's life, God filtered out everything else and revealed to me what matters most in life was in that elevator with me: God and my family.

Through this experience and others, God led me to renew my commitment for living the kind of normal life He intends for me. When it is all said and done, it won't really matter how much money any of us made, how much fun we had, or what level of worldly success we achieved. What will truly matter is what we did with our normal life and how we nurtured our most important relationships.

> *Unless the LORD builds the house, its builders labor in vain. Unless the LORD watches over the city, the guards stand watch in vain. In vain you rise early and stay up late, toiling for food to eat—for he grants sleep to those he loves. Children are a heritage from the LORD, offspring a reward from him* (Ps. 127:1-3, TNIV).

From Gracyn's Heart...

In the hospital everything was so different. What I wanted more than anything was for everything to be like it was before I got sick. I wanted it to be normal again. A lot of times it felt like I'd never be normal again. I feared I would never get out of the hospital or get to do the things I love to do again. My mom and dad would always tell me I would be normal, but sometimes I really needed to pray hard in order to believe it.

Now I am way more thankful for my normal life. Usually I don't think about the normal things and how important they are, because I am all busy and stuff. Now I stop and think a lot about how thankful I am to have family and friends, to get to play, and go to church, and do all the normal things I did before. I really don't want to be treated differently—like I had a big problem or anything. While my friends and family were so glad to see me and have me back, they don't treat me any differently than they did before I was in the hospital. I am so happy about that.

While I used to pray a lot, most of the times when I prayed I would make requests to God for things I wanted. Now when I pray I am way more thankful than I used to be. Instead of just asking for things I want, now I always thank God for what He has given me. I think it is really important for me to truly mean what I say to God. I am so thankful for all He has done for me and the normal life He has given me.

CHAPTER
9

WHEN THE WAIT
IS NEARLY OVER

Prior to Gracyn's Berlin Heart® surgery, I struggled to accept the possibility she may need a heart transplant. With every ounce of my being, I prayed for God to work the miracle of all miracles by healing her own heart. In retrospect, I was crying out for a divine miracle. However, in my limited understanding, I was placing finite parameters around what God was going to do. In truth, I was pleading for a miracle defined by my standards and fears, instead of fully trusting in God's perfect plan.

I'm sure God smiled as I begged and bargained for things that were not in His plan or what was truly needed. Eventually, I caught on to trust Him and walk by faith, rather than by my short sight. While knowing God alone is sovereign, it took a while for me to realize He desired to provide infinitely more than I could have hoped for or imagined.

Handling the Worst-Case News

As we waited anxiously with some close friends and family the night of the Berlin Heart® surgery, Dr. Byrne, a genetic heart specialist who had been involved in the surgery, introduced himself to us. He reported all was going fine, although he was totally shocked at how damaged Gracyn's heart was. After seeing her heart for the first time, the team questioned whether a virus could have done that much damage in such a short time frame. He said it was a miracle she was still alive. Even though the Berlin Heart® surgery was progressing so well, it was only going to do the job of sustaining her life for a time, not healing her heart. This doctor believed Gracyn definitely would need a heart transplant.

As the alarming news settled in, we huddled together and I began to pray. I honestly cannot recall a single word from that prayer. However, I can clearly remember the first words out of Robin's mouth as she followed me in praying aloud that night: "Father, we don't understand any of this, but we know You are in control. As a mother, I find it so hard to come to grips with the fact that another mother and a precious family somewhere are going to lose a child so that Gracyn can receive a new heart. Lord, I pray for that mother and her family. I pray for their peace and comfort. I pray You will give them strength and shower them with Your love when it is time they mourn their loss. And, I pray for that sweet child who will be giving a heart to Gracyn. Please wrap him or her in Your loving arms."

Our eyes welled up in tears as we began to pray for a family we did not know. Our hearts were heavy for this family who would gener-ously allow their child's organs to be donated so that others could live. We do not know who they are, but we continue praying for them. We cannot begin to express our feelings of gratitude for their incredible gift.

From the moment we began to explain Gracyn's heart situation with her, she amazed us with the things that would come out of her mouth. On January 2—the first day she could speak after her Berlin Heart® surgery—when she first heard of her need for a new heart, she responded, "God has a plan for me. I am walking on His path. He has saved me. I am one of His miracles."

The next morning she motioned for me to come close. Something heavy was on her mind. Still laboring deeply just to utter a few words, she whispered this question in my ear, "Daddy, will the new heart I get love Jesus like the heart I have now does?"

I explained to Gracyn the difference between a physical heart that sustains a person's life for a time and a spiritual heart, also known as a person's soul, which is our life and lasts for eternity. We began praying for God to provide a new heart to sustain her life—a new, physical heart that would beat in step with her spiritual heart, which beats so strongly for Jesus.

To help us understand what to expect when a donor heart might become available, the transplant team at Shands described what transpires on the day of transplant. They shared stories of how no one could know how long one might wait for that day to come. We listened intently as they described the excitement of when the day finally comes. Usually, the heart would come from somewhere nearby as they liked to work within a four-hour time window from donor to transplant patient. They told us of organs being transported by helicopters flying from one hospital to Shands or by helicopters flying from a hospital to an airport for a private jet to transport the organ to another helicopter that would deliver the organ to Shands…all while the clock was ticking. It sounded so exciting. And so scary.

The transplant team went on to explain how transplant coordinators would send out offers for organs as they became available. Those offers then would be evaluated by our team to determine potential match and probability for success. We received many medical lessons about matching of antibodies and antigens, blood type, size, and many other factors that would be taken into account.

While all of this was overwhelming, God had granted us peace. We knew we had some of the best physicians in the country on our side. We also knew only God could orchestrate this process and provide the heart He had chosen for our daughter. Patiently and optimistically, we waited and trusted God to provide. However, as the month of April came, we all were growing increasingly weary day by day. Each day seemed to pass by slower than before, even though we felt as though God was up to something.

FROM MY JOURNAL…

Saturday, April 4, 2009

The boys arrived around noon, and Gracyn started feeling poorly again. It is emotionally taxing for her to watch her brothers tearing around and having fun. She wants so desperately to be freed from the machine that is holding her back but, at the same time, keeping her alive. Complaining of nausea and headache, she rested most of the afternoon. We suspect the emotional pain also leads to some physical pain.

Today we prayed continually for strength. We prayed for the Lord to lift Gracyn from feelings of despair. He is with her and has a plan. Gracyn knows this. Her prayers help solidify her belief and fortify her faith. While this is so tough, she is tougher because she trusts in God and is confident in Him to carry her through. Keep praying. We know God is up to something and are waiting to see how His plan plays out.

So do not throw away your confidence; it will be richly rewarded. You need to persevere so that when you have done the will of God, you will receive what he has promised. (Heb. 10:35-36)

Sometimes we got antsy. Yet, we never really questioned why this was taking so long. A couple times our doctors told us they had passed on potential hearts for one reason or another. While this was disappointing, we were never discouraged. We believed God would provide the perfect heart in His perfect timing. We continued to live with the constant hope that today would be the day.

LIVING BETWEEN HOPE AND DISAPPOINTMENT

As we reached the fourth month of hospital confinement, we had become accustomed to our hope being dampened by still another day of waiting. We did everything possible to not dwell on the negative or give into disappointment and exhaustion. We were trying diligently to live meaningful, joy-filled lives.

Another holiday, Easter, rolled around. We determined to cele-brate that special holiday with a family slumber party in Gracyn's hospital room…

FROM MY JOURNAL…

Saturday, April 11, 2009

"Are you guys glad you're spending the night in the hospital tonight?" I overheard Gracyn quiz her brothers.

They both responded with a hearty "Yes!"

"I'm glad, too, because it will be nice to wake up on Easter morning with my family here with me."

Gracyn is thankful that God allowed her life to be saved back on Christmas day and very happy that she is healthy enough now to spend Easter with her family. She says it doesn't matter where we are as long as we are together as a family.

Please keep praying for a physical heart that will be as healthy as Gracyn's spiritual heart is. While spending Easter in a pediatric intensive care unit would certainly not be our own choice, it is, indeed, where God has us right now. So, tonight and tomorrow we will celebrate!

We celebrated that Easter as best we could…with an egg hunt in the PICU, homemade cinnamon rolls for breakfast, and Robin's famous enchiladas and chocolate sheet cake for lunch. Despite our surroundings, we truly enjoyed our special time together as a family.

This was an Easter we will always remember. We ate well, laughed a lot, and praised the Lord for His victory over sin and death.

As the day drew to a close, a battle with disappointment was building inside of me. Secretly, I had hoped God would deliver a heart for Gracyn on Easter. After all, she was admitted to the hospital on Christmas Eve. It seemed to me Easter Sunday would be the perfect day for her heart to come. But it didn't happen.

On Monday evening while driving home with Cole and Brooks, I was trying hard not to show my disappointment. But I was feeling it. The ride home was uncommonly quiet. The boys passed the time playing games on their portable game devices. I, grieving for Gracyn and feeling sorry for myself, drove in silence.

When we were at home, the boys wanted the three of us to sleep in the same room together. I crashed on my bed and the boys made themselves comfortable on my bedroom floor. Around 4:00 a.m. (Tuesday morning) I awoke and was unable to go back to sleep. Not sure what was happening, I had an intense feeling something serious was going on. Feeling that way, it was impossible for me to remain in bed. In the still of the night, I found myself wondering aimlessly around the house.

Upon reaching the kitchen, I could not contain the emotions any longer. I sprawled out on our kitchen counter and had it all out with God. Confessing my disappointment and proclaiming my weariness, I cried out for God to provide Gracyn with a new heart soon. I begged, attempted to bargain, and poured out my heart in desperation well into the morning.

I cringed as the sun came up. It had been a rough night. I felt a bit like Jacob, the Old Testament patriarch who had spent an evening wrestling with God. My back was sore. My body was exhausted. Yet, a new sense of confidence was radiating in my spirit. God had again reminded me this battle we were facing was not ours but His. He was in control and would reveal His perfect plan in His perfect timing. My night had been restless, but the new day brought with it a deep peace directly from God.

Back in Gainesville, Robin and Gracyn were up to their normal hospital routines. Gracyn got together with another patient, Cat, who was recovering nicely from a heart-and-lung-transplant. It had been such a blessing for our family to observe the transplant process Cat and her family had gone through. They had waited eleven months before Cat had received her new organs. Getting to know them helped prepare us for the day when Gracyn would receive her new heart. Plus, the two girls had some fun times together. That day they really laughed.

FROM GRACYN'S JOURNAL...

Tuesday, April 14, 2009

After walking around for a while, Mom and I decided to sing some karaoke. Cat was walking around the PICU and came by my room. Before you knew it, Cat and I were singing Hannah Montana while Mom and Nurse Monica were the back-up singers/dancers. Almost instantly, we had a crowd outside my door. Cat and I had on sunglasses and a hat with the music playing really loud. After Cat and I stopped singing, Mom, Monica, and Cat's grandma were dancing to the

Macarena while Cat and I stood there telling them how weird they looked. That was really fun.

Please pray that I will get my new heart soon. Also, pray that I can go home really soon. Thank you for praying. God loves you, and so do I.

That night, as Gracyn was getting ready to sleep, she and Robin discussed how they both had a feeling she would not be waiting much longer. Again, they laughed about the fun they had earlier and marveled at how well Cat was recovering and how healthy she seemed after her transplant. They fell asleep still waiting…perhaps a bit more expectantly than in the past.

REFLECTION:
Accept God's timing is perfect.

Looking back on all we had to endure, I can see there was a Master process in place. We all needed time to recover from Gracyn's near-death experience. We needed time to prepare for what God had in store. It took time for us to accept the fact our daughter would need a heart transplant. It took time for Gracyn to learn how to properly take medicine and prepare for a life as a transplant recipient. It took time for our family to learn how to work through all this together. Observing Cat and her family go through the transplant process helped prepare us for when our time would come.

We would journal nightly about our experiences on the Caring Bridge website and would be overwhelmed to read of all the people— over a half million hits—following our story. Reading accounts of how God was using Gracyn's story to impact thousands of people all over the world was completely humbling. We know journaling our story for all those months was also a part of God's plan. A friend pointed out the significance of our family's writing about Gracyn's story: "How astonishing it is that while thousands are praying for Gracyn's heart to be healed, thousands of hearts are actually being healed by God."

In those early morning hours, I had cried out to God from my kitchen. I knew He had a plan. I knew it without a shadow of a doubt. He could be counted on to do what was best for our family. He would fulfill His perfect will for our lives. And the lives of many others. Though worn out from the process, I knew He was with us.

> *Be strong and courageous. Do not be afraid or terrified…for the LORD your God goes with you; he will never leave you nor forsake you.* (Deut. 31:6)

FROM GRACYN'S HEART...

When Mom first told me I would need a heart transplant, I really didn't understand as I was on so many medicines that were affecting my mind. Eventually I came to understand I would need a new heart. We still prayed for God to heal my own heart because we knew He could do it if that was His plan. We also prayed for a perfect heart for a transplant if that was going to be His plan.

Before this happened to me, the only thing I knew about heart transplants was when I had watched a movie called the *Christmas Shoes*, in which a lady dies while she is waiting for a heart to come. That movie was really sad. I know a lot of people die because they have to wait too long for donor organs. I hope a lot more people will sign up to be organ donors so more lives, like mine, can be saved.

Sometimes I was scared that maybe the new heart wouldn't work right. They told me that it could work out great, and that I could be totally normal again. However, I couldn't know for sure if that would happen with me.

I prayed a lot for God to provide the perfect heart for me in His perfect timing. I knew I could depend on God. Because I trusted in Him, He gave me peace.

CHAPTER 10

WHEN THE DAY FINALLY COMES

THE MORNING OF WEDNESDAY, April 15, 2009, started out like any other normal day. I woke up my sons and prepared them a gourmet breakfast of cereal and milk. With their mom in Gainesville, their clothes may have been a bit wrinkled and their hair not as neatly combed as normal, but I did get them to school on time. As they scurried off to their classrooms, I smiled. *God, thank You for my children!* Spending this time at home with them was critical for their emotional well being and such a blessing to me. I prayed that God would bring Gracyn and Robin home to join us soon.

I headed to the office for a couple of scheduled meetings. The only thing out of the ordinary was when I realized it was income tax day. Thank goodness my extension already had been filed! It felt like it was going to be a good day.

LIFE CHANGED IN AN INSTANT

Shortly after 8:00 a.m. my cell phone rang. Upon answering I could hear Robin crying on the other end. Instinctively, I feared something terrible must have occurred.

"What happened? Is everything OK?" I asked while growing somewhat frenzied.

Teeming with emotion, Robin exclaimed, "They think they've found a heart for Gracyn! There are a few things they are still confirming, but it looks like a great match!"

Those highly anticipated words spurred feelings I had never experienced. I was elated while concerned, relieved but anxious, thrilled yet terrified. Not knowing how to take it, I eventually did what all good husbands do: I asked my wife what to do next. Robin told me to pick up the boys and head to Gainesville.

On my way back to the school, I ran into my church and quickly gathered some pastors to pray. Everyone was rejoicing with me. Then I swung by the school and picked up my boys. It was so touching to witness my boys proudly share the good news with their classmates. They were thrilled to be heading to Gainesville to see their sister prior to her heart transplant.

Our day had finally arrived! I honestly do not remember the drive up to Shands. It is as if we just somehow mysteriously arrived. When we got to the hospital, the three of us raced up to the tenth floor to see Gracyn.

Gracyn was glowing as she shared what had been happening that morning. She told us she had an unmistakable feeling something good was going to happen when she awoke that morning. She said her feeling started to be confirmed when her nurse did not bring her breakfast that morning. (Usually the first task of the day was to force some food on Gracyn before her medicine…but not this morning.) Gracyn grew even more suspicious when she noticed through the window Robin in deep conversation with Dr. Wise Eyes. She wondered why her mom had not even popped her head in the door to say good morning.

While she waited for her mom, Gracyn started doing her schoolwork. Eventually Robin entered the room. Robin said that she was immediately taken aback by the brilliance of the sun shining through the window, illuminating the beauty of our little girl as she sat quietly on the couch studying her schoolwork. They hugged as Robin, in an attempt to act as if all was normal, made small talk. Gracyn says she knew better.

When Robin finally informed her that this was the big day, Gracyn said she honestly was not surprised. She just knew it was the day. They celebrated and prayed together. God's perfect time finally had arrived!

FROM ROBIN'S JOURNAL...

Wednesday, April 15, 2009

Praise God from whom all blessings flow! We just heard this morning a heart has become available for Gracyn. Praise You, Jesus! Her surgery will be around 5:00 p.m., but in hospital time that may mean 7:00 p.m. or even later. Who knows?

They are leaving soon to get the organ and bring it here. Please pray for the family of this teenage boy. They have lost their child today. Thank You, Father, for their gift of life to us.

Just last night, Gray and I were talking. I told her I felt it was soon, very soon. I spoke with the Lord last Saturday and told Him I knew He wasn't healing Gracyn on Easter. I was fine with that (although it would've been very cool). I said, "Can it maybe be Monday, Tuesday, Wednesday, Thursday, or Friday? I'll take any of those, Lord." And, what do you know, today is the day!

As the boys and I walked down the hall of the PICU, we could feel the excitement in the air before we even made it to Gracyn's room. It was a beautiful thing to observe and feel the mood of the caregivers on a transplant day. Their enthusiasm was encouraging as they congratulated us on the arrival of this big day.

Days like this are what these very special people live for. Many of them had become like family to us. I will never again look at another medical professional—whether nurse, doctor, surgeon, respiratory therapist, administrator, and so on—without a deep sense of heartfelt gratitude for what they do. These people are true heroes!

LIFE PREPARED BY FAITH

It was truly amazing to observe Gracyn's demeanor as we awaited her surgery. It was she who in a few short hours would be put under anesthesia and have her chest opened. It was she who would have her heart removed and replaced with a new organ. It was she who would face weeks of recovery, months of rehab, and a lifetime of medication as a transplant recipient. Yet, it was she who seemed most cool, calm, and confident about what she would soon be facing. With such courageous faith my little girl has been blessed!

But Jesus called the children to him and said, "Let the little chil-
dren come to me, and do not hinder them, for the kingdom of God
belongs to such as these. I tell you the truth, anyone who will not
receive the kingdom of God like a little child will never enter it."
(Luke 18:16-17)

Because of her faith in God, Gracyn handled more than we ever
would have thought a child could handle. Early in Gracyn's illness,
we experienced the usual process of doctors sharing updates with
parents away from earshot of the child. Gracyn did not want this
and asked to be involved in these conversations. Our medical team
came to know that whatever they had to share with Robin and me
they also could share with Gracyn.

Due to the knowledge and skill of our surgeons, the advances in
medical technology, and post-surgery treatment, heart transplants
have become highly successful procedures. Of course, there are still
many risks. Prior to surgery, many of these risks had to be spelled
out and then consent given to proceed. After hearing of these risks—
including the possibility that, at the last moment, the heart may
be determined unusable or her body may reject the organ—Gracyn
maintained her courage and confidence. I will never forget her pre-
surgery prayer: "*Dear God, thank You that You may have provided a*
new heart for me. I pray that the surgery will go well and that You will
heal me. But even if it doesn't work out the way I want it to, I'm still
going to trust You!"

Oh, the faith of a child! I have never been more humbled or
proud to be known as Gracyn's father. The Lord had so effectively
used this journey to fortify her faith and to escalate our own faith.

After all this time of waiting, God had made all of us ready for this special day.

It felt like we were in a parade as the hall of the PICU lined with encouragers. Gracyn took it all in stride. She hugged and high-fived many as she made her way to the operating room (OR). Emotions and anxiety were escalating.

Again, God provided His indescribable peace. I knew we had the best surgeons and medical team available. As hard as it was to watch my little girl step through those operating room doors, I was comforted knowing she was firmly in God's omnipotent hands.

FROM ROBIN'S JOURNAL...

Wednesday, April 15, 2009, 7:37 p.m.

Around 6:00 p.m., we all walked down to the OR with Gray. She walked the whole way. (They had her bed with us in case she wanted to lie down.) Once we reached the doors to the OR, our family said our goodbyes. Then our doctors surprised us by saying one of us could go in with her. Lucky me! I put on a monkey suit and in I went. Gray was fearless! She casually walked into her OR and sat on the table. They had four flat-screens in the OR, all tuned in to the Disney channel. (Cool.) Good for distraction. They gave her the "good stuff"...and, before you knew it, she was out.

Please continue to pray for the nurses and doctors over the next few hours.

They will update us every so often. When they do, I'll post it. All glory be to God!

While Gracyn was in surgery, we had some good friends and family hang out with us. We anxiously awaited news from the OR. There was not much we could do or felt like doing. When we decided that having Cole and Brooks wait with us through the night was not the best idea, our neighbors took them home to Orlando.

Around 7:30 p.m. they began to open her chest in preparation for the heart to arrive. Sometime around 10:00 p.m. we received an update that she was on the heart-and-lung-bypass machine and all was well as the team continued to await the arrival of the heart.

Both Robin and I were flushed with emotion at the sound of a helicopter landing on the roof around 10:30 p.m. We were never told this was it, but we both felt the sound of that helicopter signaling the arrival of our daughter's new heart. Robin and I held each other and prayed quietly.

Around 2:45 a.m. we were informed the transplant had gone well and the new heart was beating strongly. There was some internal bleeding going on, but nothing about which to be concerned.

At 3:30 a.m. Dr. "Wise Eyes" emerged. He reported that the surgery had gone very well. The new heart was a bit larger than the old one. However, since her old heart had swollen so large, it had created enough space in the chest cavity for a snug, yet perfect, fit. Dr Bleiweis informed us that usually when they remove a patient's native heart it beats for a while before it eventually stops. This was not the case with Gracyn's heart. It was totally still and lifeless. Thankfully, this new heart was very healthy and everything our surgeon had hoped it would be. What a miracle we were experiencing!

Hoping to catch a few hours rest, Robin and I retired to our apartment around 5:00 a.m. We expected Gray to be out for most of the day. However, around 8:00 a.m. Robin could not resist checking in with the nurse on duty. Surprisingly, Gray was already coming to. We hurriedly returned to be by our girl!

Recovery from major surgery is a slow and painful process. In our case, we were veterans since we already had been through a prior recovery period with Gracyn. While it was comforting for us to know what to expect, it was difficult for Gracyn as she already knew the pain and struggle she would be facing.

FROM MY JOURNAL…

Thursday, April 16, 2009

Gray is doing great this morning. She is responding well and could possibly come off the ventilator this afternoon. She really wants to get that breathing tube out of her throat. At one point she motioned as if wanting something. So Robin held a dry erase board in front of her. Gracyn wrote the word "chocolate."

Dr. Wise Eyes told us her new heart is a really strong one. It is bigger than her last heart, so high blood pressure was a concern. However, so far, it has not been a problem. They have already backed off the blood pressure medicine.

There are so many things being monitored right now. Please, pray for quick healing so they can take her off drip lines, remove chest drain tubes, and take her off the ventilator. More than anything else, pray that her body will not reject her new heart. Thanks for all the

prayers and support. We will continue to update you as
we learn more.

As the hours passed, Gracyn's condition improved nicely. Dr.
Bleiweis told us everything was going remarkably well, but that he had
come to expect the remarkable when dealing with Gracyn. He confided
that Gracyn was very special to him as her personality reminded him
much of his own teenage daughter. Robin and I had really grown to
respect and admire this exceptional man and gifted surgeon whom
God had used to save so many children's lives, including Gracyn's.
It was through his skillful hands that God had worked this powerful
miracle and through his compassionate care that God had given us
such peace and confidence while we waited. We were thankful to cele-
brate the success of Gracyn's surgery with him.

As the medications wore off, Gracyn became more aware of
the pain but also aware that her surgery had gone well. Before the
surgery, when she was told she would not be able to talk when she
first woke up, Gracyn had asked us to make sure to point out she
was no longer hooked up to the Berlin Heart®. As she came to, that
was the first thing we did. She was thrilled to no longer have to rely
on a machine!

To our surprise, Tim Tebow, the quarterback, and Urban Meyer,
the head coach, for the Florida Gators, stopped by that evening and
visited with Gracyn. We told them she was not yet a big-time Gator
fan but that she was indeed a big-time Jesus fan. Robin played a
video for them of Gracyn's singing the song she wrote entitled *I Love
You More*. They were both really amazed by her and her great faith.

REFLECTION: Live life prepared.

That evening, as my daughter slept soundly with a new miracle beating in her chest, all that had transpired over the past twenty-four hours flashed through my mind. What a day it had been! I became more acutely aware of how well God had prepared us for this big day.

I realized that we had not instantly found the kind of faith we needed to deal with all of this. That faith had been developing and growing in our lives over many years. It was in the crises and struggles where the kind of faith "that can move a mountain" (Matt. 17:20) was revealed in our lives. Through our relationship with Christ, we began to take God at His Word and trust Him more than anyone or anything as we learned to "live by faith, not by sight" (2 Cor. 5:7). God had empowered us through this faith in Him every time we needed it. He was faithful and true. By following His plan for our lives, the Lord truly had prepared us for all that we faced.

Prior to Gracyn's illness, I had written a book called *SHINE: Five Empowering Principles for a Rewarding Life.* At the time, I felt God had me write that book to inspire people to live lives where the power of Christ's light can clearly be seen shining in and through them. Gazing at Gracyn in her hospital bed that evening, I realized the true purpose in writing that book was to prepare my family and me for this tough journey. Through this experience, I've learned God's Light will shine most brightly in us if we trust Him while walking through the darkest, most difficult times. Our faith is not as impactful when we shout it from the mountaintops as it is when we quietly allow it to guide us through the valleys. Genuine faith should not reflect us. It should reflect the One in whom our faith is placed.

Through the heartfelt mercies of our God, God's Sunrise will break in upon us, shining on those in the darkness, those sitting in the shadow of death, then showing us the way, one foot at a time, down the path of peace. (Luke 1: 78-79 msg).

From Gracyn's Heart...

When I woke up on April 15, I just knew it was the day. When my mom told me I would be getting a new heart, I wasn't surprised, just really excited and happy. I was pretty hyper too.

I speed-walked around the PICU about fifteen times to burn off some energy. All my nurses were really happy. Even some of the real serious doctors in the white coats, who usually didn't talk much, were all happy and congratulating me.

During the day, I started getting a little worried and scared. I knew a lot of things could go wrong and did not want any of these to happen to me. Also, going in for surgery can be pretty scary. However, when it was time to go in, we prayed, and I knew everything was going to go well. I wasn't worried because I knew God was in control.

I never thought I would say this, but it was actually good that I had to wait so long. First, I got to know all my doctors and nurses really well. I knew they were going to take great care of me. It also gave me time to get real healthy so I could recover well from surgery. While I was in the hospital, I really grew close to God. He got me ready so that when the day finally came I knew I could trust Him to get me through it.

PART FOUR

FINDING PURPOSE

For video, pictures, and interviews that relate to Part Four, go to www.gracyn.org.

CHAPTER 11

WHEN YOUR NEW NORMAL INCLUDES STORMS

THERE ARE THREE TYPES of people in the world: those who are going through a storm, those who are coming out of a storm, and those who are about to enter a storm. As much as we would all like to avoid the storms in life, no one is exempt from them.[2] Our journey with Gracyn proved storms are to be expected and will be encountered continually.

After dealing with the turbulence of one storm, we would find ourselves facing the volatility of another. The brilliant elation of the heart transplant gradually turned into the stormy reality of a difficult recovery period.

LIFE POST-OP

Worse than being in the center of the storm was watching our daughter endure many tough days during the transplant-recovery

---

2 Source unknown.

phase. As a transplant patient, Gracyn was prescribed strong anti-rejection drugs, which, by design, would suppress her body's immune system. While this is necessary to fend off rejection, it also made her much more susceptible to the dangers of infection. (It's an ongoing risk with which she is learning to live.)

Gracyn weathered her post-op storms pretty well. As her post-op days passed, we were blown away by her will and tenacity. Robin and I would wince as she bravely endured the excruciating pain of bandage changes, suture and chest tube removal, massive doses of medications, constant probing and testing, and intense physical rehab. One of the toughest challenges was post-op depression, which resulted from the heavy doses and harsh side effects of her medications.

FROM ROBIN'S JOURNAL...

Monday, April 20, 2009

Up-down, down-up, backwards-forward! Eventually we'll figure out all the meds. The whole blood pressure thing is crazy. I know the doctors are frustrated too. These things take time to work out.

At times today I felt sad because Gray was seemingly "off in another world." Her attitude most of the day was foreign to me. It's hard as a mom to watch this, although I know it's only from the meds and certainly the life-changing journey she's been on. She will settle into her old self soon.

> One of my favorite things to do as a mom is to
> comfort my children when they're in pain, hurting,
> or in need. This is not possible right now, as Gray is
> withdrawn and moody. I drew comfort from asking the
> medical team questions and learning more about what
> to expect in our situation. We're taking it one day at a
> time.

Gracyn fought valiantly. As the medical team slowly began cutting back on some of her meds, Gracyn's cheery personality began returning as well. Her determination propelled her to sit up longer than asked to, to walk one more lap around the PICU than expected, and to wow her respiratory therapists with her breathing exercises. Each challenge was met and conquered beyond expectations.

Ten days after her transplant, Gracyn was thrilled to finally be able to take a shower. Unencumbered by wires, tubes, or monitors, she skipped briskly through the hallway and cheerfully sang, "I'm free, free at last!" Then, as the water cascaded over her, she ecstatically proclaimed, "I am so happy!"

By Sunday, since all was going well, it finally appeared the time had come for Gracyn to check out of the hospital. Arrangements would be made the next morning for her discharge. Gracyn was elated. Our whole family was thrilled. Cole and Brooks had been up in Gainesville with us all weekend. The next day was such a big day. We agreed to let them skip school that Monday so we could enjoy the ride home together.

FROM BROOKS'S AND GRACYN'S JOURNALS...

Sunday, April 26, 2009, 9:35 p.m.

Hello, everybody! This is Brooks. I am glad it is the last night for Gracyn to be in the hospital. She is coming home tomorrow. We will be having so much fun when she gets home. It has been so hard not having my sister at home. But now it is finally time for her to come home. God has taken care of her this whole time. I am so happy He takes care of us. I am so glad our whole family will be together again at home.

Hello, everybody! This is Gracyn. I am glad Brooks wrote to you while I took my medicine. I have waited for this day for four months. Some days I felt like it would never get here. This has been, and probably will be, the hardest time of my life. I could not have done it without my Lord and Savior Jesus Christ. He has given me strength through all of it...and I know He will continue to give me strength for the rest of my life. Some days when I was in so much pain and wanted to be home, Mom and Dad would always say to have faith in Him and that He would bring me home some day. Some days when I wanted it to hurry up—because it seemed like it was taking so long—I had to learn to believe in God's perfect timing. Now I know His timing is just right!

While the forecast for the day of Gracyn's homecoming was sunny and warm, another unexpected storm blew in. Throughout that highly anticipated final night, an irregular heartbeat began to reveal itself. Considering all Gracyn had already endured, this storm hit at what seemed the worst time and reached its pinnacle the next morning when we had to inform Gracyn she would not be going home as planned.

Four months of anticipation flooded in on her. She initially could not be consoled. Weeping, she began apologizing for being in the hospital for so long. She was sorry for messing up our lives. She wondered how we still could love her when she was stuck in a hospital all this time. She needed to release it all.

The emotional meltdown was heartbreaking. Our whole family was disappointed. All we could do was tell her how much we loved her and remind her God loves her even more.

As the torrents of tears raged, I was reminded there was only one place true shelter could be found:

> *He who dwells in the shelter of the Most High will rest in the shadow of the Almighty. I will say of the LORD, "He is my refuge and my fortress, my God, in whom I trust."* (Ps. 91:1-2)

We learned from a biopsy that a mild case of rejection was indeed taking place. This required a few more days of strong, anti-rejection medication. It was so hard for Gracyn to accept this disappointing setback. I cannot explain adequately the pain I felt watching my child curl up in utter sadness on her hospital bed as she sobbed uncontrollably. I also cannot begin to express the sheer joy and pride I felt when she eventually accepted this setback as just another obstacle to be overcome while trusting in God's plan to carry her through. God helped us weather yet another storm.

One afternoon as we continued our waiting, we were given an opportunity to view Gracyn's native heart. They brought it up from the lab and showed us the hole in the bottom of her left atrium where one of the Berlin tubes had been inserted. It was fascinating. This opportunity allowed Gracyn to join a very rare fraternity of individuals who have held their own heart in their hands. When asked what she thought of holding her own heart, she replied, "I never thought my heart would look so much like chicken."

LIFE "BACK TO NORMAL"

Finally, on May 1, we were cleared to check out of Shands Hospital. It was an emotional day as we said our goodbyes and thanked our caregivers. Numerous nurses, through tears, hugged Gray and thanked her for changing their lives.

The chief cardiologist, Dr. Fricker, thanked me. I was shocked someone for whom I was so thankful would be thanking me. He expressed appreciation for the powerful impact Gracyn and our family had made on the tenth floor. I explained we never tried to make an impact. We just trusted God. If any impact had been made, it was God's doing. He concurred and responded he was thankful for the faith they had all seen lived out by our family over the past months.

Gracyn was so excited to actually sit in a car for the first time in nearly five months. (It's amazing how the simplest things in life are missed when we can't do them for a while.) As we drove off, I noticed the Life-Flight helicopter approaching the hospital roof for a landing. It was on that same roof Gracyn had arrived so many nights ago with such a slim chance of survival. While mentally reliving our incredible journey over the past months, I overheard Gracyn say, "Someday I'd like to see what Gainesville really looks like…but not now. Right now, I just want to go home!" Overjoyed by the priceless gift we had been given, it was the happiest drive our family has ever taken.

Gracyn beamed as we pulled into our neighborhood. Our neighbors had hung red hearts on every trunk of our tree-lined street. Our yellow lab, Biscuit, eagerly met us at the front door.

Without ceremony, Gracyn walked around the house to confirm all was still normal. Once she was satisfied, we all hugged each other and thanked God for His incredible blessings.

Later that afternoon, our cul-de-sac filled with friends, classmates, neighbors, acquaintances, and local police. (The police were curious as to what had drawn so many cars to our community and so many people to our street.) Together we sang songs of praise, prayed, and simply rejoiced in all that our God and Healer had done for us!

The next few days were precious. Simple things like gathering around our kitchen island to share a meal, taking a walk around the block, or just playing in our yard all seemed so much more enjoyable than ever before. Gracyn was thrilled to be home and enjoying her new "normal."

Even our family dog, Biscuit, seemed happier now that our family was reunited back home. One night Gracyn asked if I could have Biscuit share his thoughts in the Caring Bridge journal. At that point Gracyn was getting everything she asked for, so naturally I obliged.

From Biscuit's journal…

Friday, May 2, 2009

Hi, everybody! Biscuit, the family dog, here. The most amazing thing happened yesterday. My best friend came back home. I'm not sure how long she was gone, but it seemed like forever. (Don't tell anybody, but I used to lose my self-control and wander the neighborhood looking for her.) Now I have peace in knowing right where she is. It is so good having the whole family back together again. Last night when they put me to bed, I was overjoyed to hear my favorite sound in the whole world. Yup, my best girl was sweetly singing me to sleep just like she used to. It doesn't get much better than that. There is just so much—arf!—to be thankful for!

For a time the storms subsided. Our family experienced a high point in our journey, although there were many challenges to come. As time passed, we began to understand some of the hurts and struggles our sons had endured over the time of Gracyn's illness. Robin, especially, mourned for the time away from them and the deep wounds this had apparently caused for our boys. Even though she had been supermom in everyone's book, Robin felt guilt about the pain our sons were dealing with.

Statistics show that traumatic experiences like Gracyn's illness take a great toll on families and marriages. For months, Robin and I had been so focused on caring for Gracyn we subsequently had ignored our relationship. We came to realize there was much healing that needed to take place in our home. The best remedy would be spending time together. Once again, God proved His timing is perfect as we had a whole summer ahead of us. With no school for the kids, we could reconnect as a family.

The months progressed. More storms raged. But we consistently found refuge together as a family in the firm foundation of our faith.

> *Therefore everyone who hears these words of mine and puts them into practice is like a wise man who built his house on the rock. The rain came down, the streams rose, and the winds blew and beat against that house; yet it did not fall, because it had its foundation on the rock."* (Matt. 7:24-25)

REFLECTION: STICK WITH THE PLAN.

I am in the construction equipment business. Needless to say, 2008 was one of the toughest years our company had ever encountered. That is, until 2009 rolled around. In the midst of our family crises, we also endured a serious business crisis.

For many months, our business had been struggling. As the CEO, I was doing my best to handle things at work while my heart was really focused on tending to Gracyn. Thankfully, God has blessed us with some outstanding folks who all rose to the occasion to take care of business.

As I settled back into my work full-time, the struggles were overwhelming. We had lost more than half our revenues in less than two years. In an effort to survive as a corporation, we were forced to painstakingly cut expenses and, to some degree, downsize. It was incredibly tough to make all of these life-impacting decisions that involved our company and the lives of employees. The gravity of it all weighed heavily on my heart and mind.

Late one evening, I was sitting around feeling sorry for myself and our company when Robin walked by. She said, "You look like a depressed dufus! What's wrong?" Talk about encouragement!

Quite honestly, that was exactly what I needed. Robin reminded me of how, at the worst moments with Gracyn, we had trusted God, and He had faithfully pulled us through. She reiterated He would do the same in our business if I would just stop acting like a dufus and trust Him. She reminded me in her lighted-hearted but seriously right-on way to stick with the plan.

Over the course of time, I've seen God's faithfulness guide our company, sustain us, and keep us out of the pit. Times are still challenging, and difficult decisions continue to loom. However, when I tell people faith will carry us through, I do so in full confidence and with fire-forged credibility.

God also guides the details of Gracyn's life as she has resumed her normal life and re-engaged in regular activities. Gracyn had studied regularly while in the hospital. With the help of a summer tutor, she was promoted and entered the fifth grade in August. As winter rolled around, Gracyn decided she wanted to resume playing basketball. She was healthy enough to return to the court on her school's fifth-grade girls' basketball team.

The first quarter of the first game did not go well. Her team trailed 6-0. As I looked over at the bench, I noticed Gracyn crying. Instinctively fearing the worst, I ran over and asked if she was OK, "Does your chest hurt? Are you feeling winded?"

"No Dad, she whimpered. "I'm just not any good anymore. Before I got sick I was good, but now I can't even make a basket."

My heart ached for her. As she was sulking, my mind flashed back to Robin's "stop acting like a dufus" conversation. Though genuinely tempted to pull that one out, I wisely took another approach with the same tact: "Remember back in the hospital when you thought you would never get out of there and that you would never get better? Remember when you would have doubts about your faith in God? Remember those few times when you didn't want to pray, didn't want to trust, and didn't want to believe? Well, the same thing is happening to you right now. But remember, you did not listen to those lies in the hospital. Instead, you listened to God's promises and, by faith, you trusted Him. You chose to listen to the Voice of Truth, not to a bunch of lies. You are a good basketball player. You will be better. You need to trust God just like you did in the hospital. Now, get out there and do your best!"

I'm proud to say that by the third quarter she was a dynamo with multiple steals, great ball-handling, and even scoring six points! Throughout the gymnasium, tears were flowing and fans cheering. We all were amazed. By the end of the season, her team won the championship game…and Gracyn led her team in scoring for that game. Again, we were in awe of God's goodness and faithfulness.

No matter what storms we may face, we have come to know, beyond a doubt, there is One who can calm any storm! We have learned we should confidently take one step at a time and, by faith, stick to the plan:

1. Know God is with you.
2. Release your burden to God.

3. Seek *what* instead of *why*.

4. Trust in God's life-changing power.

5. Believe God still works miracles.

6. Rely on God's perfect strength.

7. Recognize God's plan is worth the wait.

8. Focus on what is most important.

9. Accept God's timing is perfect.

10. Live life prepared.

CHAPTER 12

WHEN YOU BEGIN TO GRASP THE WHY

On Father's Day, June 21, 2009, our entire family was able to worship together at our church for the first time since Gracyn's illness. During the morning announcements, one of the television cameras focused on Gracyn as her return was announced. The whole congregation cheered. It was a joyous celebration.

The worship pastor came to us and quietly asked if Gracyn would like to join the praise team on stage for the closing song after the pastor's sermon. The song they would be singing was Kari Jobe's *Healer*, which was a special song to us because Gracyn had listened to that song every night in the hospital before she would go to sleep. Our pastor told Gracyn, "You don't have to worry about singing a solo or anything. You can just stand up there with the praise team."

To this Gracyn replied, "I don't mind. I'll sing!"

What our pastor didn't realize is that back in the hospital Gracyn and Robin had often discussed that someday Gracyn would sing that song in church. It is so amazing how God was orchestrating all this.

With no prior warning and with no fear, Gracyn took the stage in front of nearly four thousand worshippers. With eyes lifted heavenward, a microphone in one hand, and the other hand placed directly over her new heart, she lifted her voice in praise.

Gracyn clearly was no longer just singing a song. She was the song, a miraculous song of praise directly purposed to glorify her Healer. Not only was it the most intense moment of worship in my life, it was the greatest Father's Day gift ever!

A few weeks later, Gracyn was given the opportunity to sing that same song with Kari Jobe at one of her concerts. God has continued to give Gracyn the opportunity to sing many times for churches, charity events, school chapel services, and other venues. Oh, how my little girl loves to sing!

LIVING YOUR LIFE SONG

Some months before Gracyn's illness, she was singing a catchy tune as she walked into our room. Robin asked her where she had heard that song. "I made it up," Gracyn proclaimed.

With Robin's encouragement, she proceeded to add a couple verses to the chorus, and, eventually, had her first composition, which she entitled "I Love You More."

> *I love You more than the stars that shine on me,*
> *I love You more than the waves in the rambling seas.*
> *I love You more, Jesus, than anything;*
> *I love You more.*

A short time later, Gracyn was asked to sing this song for a chapel service at her school. After this performance, she was the talk of the school. Children asked for her autograph and proclaimed she would win American Idol someday. It was really cute.

That evening, Gracyn came downstairs after taking her shower. She talked with Robin. Gracyn told Robin she really loved singing at school and thought it was pretty cool the way the kids responded to her song. She went on to explain, "Mom, it is not my dream to be known as a great singer. I don't want the spotlight to shine on me. I just want God's light to shine through me."

Touched by the spiritual maturity of our nine-year-old daughter, Robin reminded Gracyn that God has given her a special gift and has a purpose for her to use that gift for His glory. That night, and many other times since, Gracyn has prayed for God to use her singing and songwriting for His glory.

It was within two month's time from this conversation with Robin that we nearly lost Gracyn.

FROM MY JOURNAL...

Monday, May 18, 2009

Earlier this evening, I overheard my wife and daughter singing together a song of praise. It brought me back to a not-so-distant memory. Initially, while Gracyn lay unconscious in her hospital bed with her earthly future questionable at best, Robin would sing songs of praise over her. While being kept alive by the Berlin Heart®, Gracyn slowly began to recover. I can still feel that simple sense of pure joy in hearing Gray's quiet, trembling voice join with Robin's in song.

You see, no matter the situation, they would sing continuously throughout this ordeal. Numerous times hospital staff and other parents would question how we could endure such a trial with smiles on our faces and with Robin and Gracyn singing so much of the time. My response was always simple: "They are worshiping our Creator, the One we trust to heal our daughter. Regardless of our current circumstance, He is worthy of our praise. Worship is all about Him. It is His grace that brings smiles to our faces and songs of praise to our hearts."

I can truly say that worship will never be the same for me. Now that Gracyn is home and doing so well, I continually think about her throughout the day. I think of where she's been, where she is now, and where she will someday be. Her songs fill my mind, and my heart overflows with thankfulness to our God.

At some of the most uncertain moments—times when Gracyn's life was literally hanging in the balance—Robin and I were comforted by a recurring thought: God has placed a song in Gracyn's heart and has more songs for her to sing. We had to accept the possibility that Gray's songs might be sung in Heaven, rather than here on earth. Realizing God might take her from us, we knew we could trust Him, no matter what the outcome might be.

Robin and I came to understand that true faith is not believing God will do what we want Him to do. True faith is accepting God's will regardless of what it may be. We will be eternally grateful God's plan allowed Gracyn to remain with us.

Gracyn has not stopped singing since her surgery. God continues to provide opportunities for her to sing and us to share her story. While we have been the benefactors of a great miracle, we realize the purpose of this miracle was not just to bless us but to glorify God and to draw others to Him.

Gracyn and I used to think of things we could do to spend father-daughter time together. Now we get to minister to others by sharing her story while she sings for His glory. It doesn't get much better than that!

His Purpose Revealed

The other day, I sat at our kitchen table quietly observing Gracyn as she worked on her homework. Gracyn paused, looked up, and said, "Dad, I think I know now why I had to go through such a tough time with my heart."

With anticipation for what would be revealed, I leaned in. She went on to explain, "I've always loved to sing. But, before, when I would sing, I didn't really feel anything. I was just singing because I loved to sing. Now when I sing I can feel God working in me. Now when I sing it's my way of thanking God. I can see people's lives being changed by Him while I sing. And I like that a whole lot better. I want to tell as many people as I can about the miraculous things God has done for me. My life is like His song…and I sing it for His glory!"

We always knew God had more songs for her to sing!

We know that in all things God works for the good of those who love him. He appointed them to be saved in keeping with his purpose. (Rom. 8:28 NIRV)

One morning in January, 2009, soon after coming to from her Berlin Heart® surgery, Gracyn mentioned something she said happened "while I was dead." We informed her she had been very close to dying but never actually had been dead. She had only been in a coma. Not fully agreeing with us, Gracyn went on to explain she had been in a very dark pit and could not get out. She said she was getting worried, but then Jesus pulled her out of the pit. After that happened, she said she knew she wasn't going back to the pit and was going to be OK. We gently asked her for more details of what she said had transpired. However, at that time, that is all she said.

A few days later, I was reading Psalm 40 and knew in my heart it related to Gracyn, to her story, and to her song:

> *I was patient while I waited for the Lord.*
>   *He turned to me and heard my cry for help.*
>
> *I was sliding down into the pit of death, and he pulled me out.*
>   *He brought me up out of the mud and dirt.*
>
> *He set my feet on a rock.*
>   *He gave me a firm place to stand on.*
> *He gave me a new song to sing.*
>   *It is a hymn of praise to our God.*
>
> *Many people will see what he has done and will worship him.*
>   *They will put their trust in the Lord.* (Ps. 40:1-3 NIRV)

Robin and I did not want to prod Gracyn or push her to relay more details. Yet, we were interested in hearing more about her time in the pit. Each time we would bring it up, she would always say, "That's when I was dead. I can't explain it to you, because you won't understand." For a long time we left it alone.

While writing this book, I explained the content of each chapter to Gracyn and asked her what she wanted to tell readers about that chapter in her "From Gracyn's Heart" section. For the end of this chapter I asked her if she would try once again to explain to me her account of being in the pit. She smiled and said, "Dad I told you that you just won't understand. Until you get to Heaven, you just won't get it."

I implored her to try again. This is what she told me…

From Gracyn's Heart…

"Dad, this is so hard to explain in words, but I will try. In fact, there aren't any words to describe it. The only thing I can say is you'll understand when you get to heaven. You will only know it when you feel it.

"It seemed like you and Mom left me, and you weren't coming back. That's when I ended up in the pit. The pit is scary and devastating. It is so dark and feels like everything has ended. I could feel others around me, but I couldn't see them. Nobody wanted to be in the pit. It was very gloomy. I felt like I was stuck. I knew I couldn't get out of there on my own.

"I really don't know how to say this. Suddenly, I got a deep, holy, and pure feeling. I knew God was there. The darkness tried to stay, but it faded away. It's like a light just overpowered it. I can't explain the light. It's like nothing we've seen here. It is extremely bright but not like electric light—not like what light looks like here. It's glorious and so different. The thing is you don't just see the light; you feel it…and you hear it too. It is beyond words! It is so awesome! But *awesome* is not a good enough word to describe the light.

"The light told me—not with words, but with a feeling—that I was out of the pit and not going back into the pit. I knew I didn't need to be afraid of the pit anymore. I felt God's voice and I could hear the light. His voice and His light are the same. He told me He was doing miracles…and that I was one of His miracles. It was like I wasn't really seeing with my eyes, but I could still see because seeing, hearing, and feeling are all the same. You just know things. You aren't afraid of anything anymore, and you feel totally secure.

"There may have been others there, but I didn't see them. It kind of felt like others might be there, but I'm not sure. I wasn't really thinking about others because all I could see, feel, or think about was God. I didn't have to go somewhere to worship Him because He was everywhere. I knew there was singing going on, but in Heaven you don't really sing with voices, you sing with your heart. All I could feel was that I was with God. I was safe. I knew all was good. I knew He had plans for me. I was one of His songs.

"Like I said, I really can't explain it. There just aren't words. You will know what I mean when you get to feel it someday for yourself. Heaven isn't up or down, east or west. Heaven is where Jesus is. When you are with Jesus, you are in Heaven…and nothing else matters."

Thank you, Gracyn, for helping me to understand. You've taught me more than you will ever know. You have been given an incredible gift. I love how you faithfully share your heart with others. You are a miracle!

Thank You, God, for Your miraculous plan. You sent Your Son as the perfect donor. Thank You that, through Him, we can all be given a new heart…and a new song!

> Lord my God, no one can compare with you.
> You have done many miracles.
> And you plan to do many more for us.
> There are too many of them
> for me to talk about. (Ps. 40:5 NIRV)

You Have the Power to Save a Life

THE POWER OF ORGAN and tissue donation is evidenced in the thousands of lives that are saved due to a special kind of hero— an organ and tissue donor. We are truly blessed Gracyn is one of these lives.

Transplantation has the ability to free someone from kidney dialysis, help a child walk, or even allow individuals to see their loved ones for the first time. The results are life-changing.

Unfortunately, donation does not occur nearly enough for the many in need. National research conducted by Donate Life America concluded that a majority of Americans support donation, yet few know how to designate their desire to become organ and tissue donors.

We have the power to make a difference. Please, learn the facts, make a decision, and share what you know with others.

Start now by visiting www.donatelife.net.

Gracyn knows that Romans 8:28 is true, "And we know that in all things God works for the good of those who love him, who have been called according to his purpose." He has provided Gracyn with a great purpose to touch the lives of others through her song.

If you have been touched by her story, you can play a key role in spreading this message of hope by simply telling others about it.

IF YOU'RE A FAN OF THIS BOOK, PLEASE TELL OTHERS...

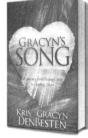

- Give *Gracyn's Song* as a gift.

- Write about *Gracyn's Song* on your website, blog, Twitter, MySpace, or Facebook page.

- Email your friends and contacts to tell them about the website: www.gracyn.org.

- Share *Gracyn's Song* with someone you know who is facing a crisis.

- Tell pastors, counselors, hospital chaplains you may know about *Gracyn's Song*.

- Talk about the story on email lists or other internet forums you frequent.

CONNECT WITH THE DENBESTEN FAMILY...

Gracyn specifically desires to help feed and educate children in Haiti, to help families who are dealing with crisis, and to support the pediatric heart programs that helped save her life. We have established an organization called Gracyn's Heart to help support some of these causes.

You can find out more about Gracyn's Heart by connecting with us at:

> **Real Life Resources**
> **4401 Vineland Road**
> **Suite A15**
> **Orlando, FL 32811**
> **Email: gracynsheart@gmail.com**
> **Website: www.gracyn.org**

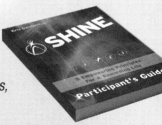